ALLERGIES AND INFECTIOUS DISEASES

TUBERCULOSIS AND MULTIDRUG-RESISTANT TUBERCULOSIS

EPIDEMIOLOGY, DIAGNOSIS, RESISTANCE MECHANISMS, TREATMENT STRATEGIES AND NOVEL DRUGS

ALLERGIES AND INFECTIOUS DISEASES

Additional books in this series can be found on Nova's website under the Series tab.

Additional e-books in this series can be found on Nova's website under the e-book tab.

PUBLIC HEALTH IN THE 21ST CENTURY

Additional books in this series can be found on Nova's website under the Series tab.

Additional e-books in this series can be found on Nova's website under the e-book tab.

ALLERGIES AND INFECTIOUS DISEASES

TUBERCULOSIS AND MULTIDRUG-RESISTANT TUBERCULOSIS

EPIDEMIOLOGY, DIAGNOSIS, RESISTANCE MECHANISMS, TREATMENT STRATEGIES AND NOVEL DRUGS

SUHAIL AHMAD
AND
EIMAN MOKADDAS

NOVA BIOMEDICAL

New York

Library of Congress Cataloging-in-Publication Data

ISBN: 978-1-62808-309-5

LCCN: 2013942218

Published by Nova Science Publishers, Inc. † New York

Contents

Preface

The worldwide incidence of tuberculosis (TB) has been declining slowly over the last few years due to increased public and private investments and joint efforts of the World Health Organization and health care systems of various countries. Despite these developments, the global burden of TB still remains enormous. With nearly 9 million active disease cases and 1.5 million deaths occurring worldwide every year, TB is a major public health issue and a leading cause of death from an infectious agent in most of the developing countries. Active TB disease in most countries is caused by *Mycobacterium tuberculosis*, an obligate human pathogen. The worldwide TB epidemic is being sustained by the increasing incidence of drug-resistant, multidrug-resistant (MDR) (resistant at least to rifampicin and isoniazid) and extensively drug-resistant (XDR) (additionally resistant to a fluoroquinolone plus kanamycin/amikacin/capreomycin) strains of *M. tuberculosis* and association of active disease with human immunodeficiency virus (HIV) coinfection or other underlying immunosuppressive conditions such as diabetes. Rapid diagnosis and drug susceptibility testing (DST) of *M. tuberculosis* strains to anti-TB drugs ensure effective treatment. Rapid molecular diagnostic and DST methods have been developed recently. Treatment of drug-susceptible TB is effective in $\geq$95% of disease cases, however, supervised therapy for $\geq$6 months is challenging. Non-adherence to treatment often results in much lower cure rates and evolution of drug-resistant strains of *M. tuberculosis* due to mutations occurring at a predictable rate in genes encoding drug targets. Drug-susceptible strains are killed while drug-resistant strains survive and multiply during inappropriate therapy. Sequential accumulation of mutations results in evolution of MDR and XDR strains of *M. tuberculosis*. Effective treatment of MDR-TB involving therapy with 5-7 less efficacious, expensive and toxic second-line/third-line drugs for $\geq$18-24 months is challenging. XDR-TB is difficult to treat even in developed countries and is virtually untreatable in developing countries. Proper management of MDR-TB/XDR-TB relies on early recognition and effective treatment of such patients. Both, low-cost, phenotypic and more expensive, rapid molecular diagnostic methods have been developed recently for identification of MDR-TB/XDR-TB strains from suspected patients and some are also now available commercially. Once identified, successful treatment of MDR-TB/XDR-TB requires supervised aggressive therapy with several (5-7) expensive, toxic and less efficacious (second-line and third-line) drugs for $\geq$24 months which complicates adherence to treatment. Effective treatment of MDR-TB/XDR-TB requires supervised therapy with appropriate drugs at specialized institutions equipped with modern facilities for rapid culture, drug susceptibility testing of MDR-TB/XDR-TB strains to second-line and third-line drugs and regular monitoring of patients for adverse drug reactions and bacteriological and clinical improvement. Some currently existing drugs and several new drugs, some with novel mode of action, are in various stages of clinical development to improve the outcome of MDR-TB/XDR-TB. Some of these drugs are currently in phase III clinical trials and Food and Drug Administration (FDA) of the United States of America has recently approved one drug (bedaquiline) for the treatment of selected MDR-TB patients. The newer agents may shorten treatment duration for drug-susceptible TB and may help in the effective treatment of MDR-TB/XDR-TB.

Suhail Ahmad and Eiman Mokaddas
Department of Microbiology,
Faculty of Medicine,
Kuwait University, Kuwait

Corresponding author:
Prof. Suhail Ahmad
Department of Microbiology
Faculty of Medicine, AMAR Health Sciences Center
Kuwait University, P. O. Box 24923, Safat 13110
Kuwait
Email: suhail_ah@hsc.edu.kw; suhail_ah2000@yahoo.com
Tel: 00965-2463-6503; Fax: 00965-2531-8454

Chapter I

Natural History of Tuberculosis

Tuberculosis (TB) is an infectious disease with a long history. Most active TB disease cases in humans are caused by *Mycobacterium tuberculosis* while some cases are also caused by *Mycobacterium africanum* and *Mycobacterium bovis,* two of the other six species belonging to *M. tuberculosis* complex (MTBC). All MTBC members are obligate intracellular pathogens and cause TB but exhibit distinct phenotypic properties and host range [1]. They are closely related genetically and have nearly identical genome organization. The genome sequence of *M. tuberculosis* shows >99.9% similarity with *M. bovis,* the species which primarily infects cattle but can also cause TB in individuals who consume unpasteurized milk [2, 3].

Tuberculosis is one of the most common infections of human beings and a formidable public health challenge, particularly in poor and developing countries around the world. According to the surveys conducted by World Health Organization (WHO), the global incidence of TB has been declining slowly during the last 20 years, however, the global burden of TB is still enormous. The disease contributes significantly to illness and death worldwide and mainly afflicts young adults in their most productive years. Major factors sustaining the global burden of TB include increasing incidence of resistance of *M. tuberculosis* strains to the most effective (first-line) and important second-line anti-TB drugs and rising incidence of human immunodeficiency virus (HIV) infection and its association with active TB disease [4-6]. Other important factors contributing or likely to contribute to active TB disease include growing population of immunocompromised/immunosuppressed individuals, association of active disease with other underlying conditions such as diabetes mellitus, inadequate TB control/prevention programs in developing countries, active transmission in overcrowded places (such as prisons) resulting in infection and re-infection and poor case detection and cure rates in high TB burden countries [7-10].

The natural history of *M. tuberculosis* infection is quite unique. Inhalation of droplet nuclei containing few bacilli during close contact of human subjects with sputum smear-positive pulmonary TB patients (open TB) is mainly responsible for new TB infections. Studies carried out in cohorts of human subjects have shown that primary infection with *M. tuberculosis* leads to clinically active TB disease in only 5-10% of exposed individuals [11, 12]. The protective immune response mounted by other immunocompetent hosts arrests further multiplication of tubercle bacilli but complete (sterile) eradication of the pathogen is achieved in nearly 10% of the infected individuals only. In the remaining individuals, sub-optimal immune reponse, due to blunting of microbicidal mechanisms of phagocytic immune cells by *M. tuberculosis* factors, only succeeds in containment of infection as some tubercle bacilli escape killing and transform into non-replicating (dormant or latent) state in granulomatous lesions and persist [12-14].

Individuals infected with *M. tuberculosis* show differences in the innate immune responses that lead to the formation of physiologically distinct granulomatous lesions. Early stages of granuloma formation benefit *M. tuberculosis* as the tubercle bacilli multiply in infected phagocytic cells which may also transport the pathogen to other (extra-pulmonary) sites in the body [15, 16]. The eventual formation of solid granuloma due to an effective immune response walls off tubercle bacilli from the rest of the lung tissue, limits bacterial spread and provide microenvironment for interactions among immune cells and the cytokines released from these cells. Some of these lesions eliminate all bacilli (sterilizing immunity) while others only arrest growth but allow persistence of viable *M. tuberculosis* in the microenvironment (latent *M. tuberculosis* infection, latent TB) [16, 17]. The hypoxia, low pH and inhibition of respiration by nitric oxide in the microenvironment of the granuloma also induce a dormancy program regulated by DosR in *M. tuberculosis* [18]. The latent TB infection in a person without overt signs of the disease is indicated by the delayed-type hypersensitivity response to purified protein derivative prepared from culture filtrates of *M. tuberculosis* (tuberculin skin test) [7, 16].

The latent infection may remain dormant for a long time, however, *M. tuberculosis* retains the capability to resuscitate and cause active TB disease in the event of disruption of host's immune response [12, 19]. Although reactivation of latent infection can occur even decades after initial infection, a person is at a greater risk of developing active TB disease during the first two years after infection with *M. tuberculosis* [7, 12, 19]. Several factors can trigger development of active disease from reactivation of remote infection, and typically involve the weakening of the immune system [12, 19]. HIV infection is the most important risk factor for progression to active disease in adults as it causes depletion/functional abnormalities of immune cells ($CD4^+$ T cells) that are central for protection against active TB disease [4, 19]. It is estimated that ~2.2 billion people (nearly one-third of the total world population) are now latently infected with tubercle bacilli and 5%-10% of the infected individuals will eventually develop active TB disease during their life time [16, 19]. Although reactivation of latent infection is the major mechanism of active TB disease in low TB incidence countries, recent infection or re-infection is also common among high TB burden countries [7, 12]. The risk of reactivation of latent infection is much higher in human subjects with underlying immunodeficiencies, diabetes or coinfection with HIV. It is estimated that the annual risk of active TB is 5%-15% and the lifetime risk is ~50% in HIV-seropositive individuals [4, 12, 19]. The main focus of this book is accurate and early diagnosis of drug-susceptible and drug-resistant TB, effective treatment of drug-susceptible and drug-resistant active TB disease and new drugs which are in various stages of clinical development for effective treatment of drug-resistant TB and for shortening treatment duration of fully susceptible pulmonary TB, key pre-requisites for a successful global TB control in the 21st cenury. Other control measures such as diagnosis and treatment of latent tuberculosis infection and development of vaccines to control the TB epidemic are outside the scope but the reader is directed to excellent recent reviews available in the literature [12, 16, 17, 20].

Chapter II

Global Epidemiology of TB, Drug-Resistant TB, MDR-TB and XDR-TB

The WHO has conducted annual surveys for the worldwide incidence and prevalence of new and relapse cases of TB and has provided information about TB epidemic and progress in TB care and control at global, regional and country levels for the last several years. The latest report published in 2012 showed that new cases of TB are falling at a rate of 2.2% since 2010. The TB mortality rate has decreased 41% since 1990 and the world is on target to achieve the global target of a 50% reduction in mortality by 2015 [21]. The report has also shown that mortality and incidence rates are falling in all six regions of WHO and in most of 22 high TB burden countries.

Despite these positive developments, the global burden of TB still remains enormous. Recent estimates showed that there were 8.7 million incident cases of active TB disease worldwide corresponding to an estimated incidence of 125 per 100,000 population in 2011 [21]. Nearly 1.1 million (13%) of TB patients were coinfected with HIV. Most of the estimated cases in 2011 occurred in Asia (59%) and Africa (26%) while smaller proportions of cases occurred in the Eastern Mediterranean region (7.7%), the European region (4.3%) and the Region of the Americas (3%). The 22 high TB burden countries accounted for 82% of all estimated incident TB cases. The top five countries included India, China, South Africa, Indonesia and Pakistan [21]. The highest incidence rate (262 per 100,000 population) was recorded for the African region, mainly due to higher prevalence of concomitant HIV infection.

More TB patients are now being tested for HIV-coinfection, particularly in the African region. In 2011, 69% of TB patients were tested for HIV in the African region while only 3% TB patients were tested for HIV in 2004. Nearly 39% of TB cases in the African region were coinfected with HIV which accounted for 79% of all TB cases among people living with HIV worldwide [21]. The incidence rates of 28, 42, 109, 189 and 92 per 100,000 population were recorded for the Americas, European region, Eastern Mediterranean region, South-East Asia region and Western Pacific region, respectively, in 2011. Globally, a total of 12 million prevalent TB cases resulted in 1.4 million deaths in 2011 (990,000 among HIV-seronegative and 430,000 among HIV-coinfected individuals). This is the first time that the number of deaths among HIV-seronegative TB patients has fallen below 1 million individuals in recent years. These deaths also included 0.5 million women, thus making TB as one of the top killers of women worldwide [21]. Overall, there were an estimated 20 deaths per 100,000 population (including both, HIV-seronegative and HIV-coinfected individuals) in 2011.

The WHO has also carried out surveys (Global Projects on Antituberculosis Drug Resistance Surveillance) for estimating the incidence of drug resistant TB by collecting drug susceptibility testing (DST) data for first-line drugs; isoniazid (INH), rifampicin (RIF), ethambutol (EMB) and streptomycin (SM) [5, 22]. Phenotypic DST for another first-line drug, pyrazinamide (PZA) is not carried out routinely in clinical mycobacteriology laboratories as this drug is active at acidic pH which complicates susceptibility testing [23]. The two recent comprehensive reports gathered DST data from surveys or ongoing surveillance between 2002-2007 and between 2007-2010 [5, 22]. The data on new TB cases between 2002-2007 were available from 72 countries and showed that resistance to at least one anti-TB drug (defined as any resistance) among new TB cases was 11.1% (varying from 0% to 56%). The prevalence of resistance to any drug was higher than 30% in 13 countries or settings. The worldwide average for multidrug-resistant TB (MDR-TB, defined as infection with *M. tuberculosis* strains resistant at least to RIF and INH, the two most effective anti-TB drugs) was determined as 2.9%. The proportion of MDR-TB among new cases between 2007-2010 ranged from 0% to 28.9% among new TB cases. The data on previously treated TB cases were available from 66 countries and showed that resistance to at least one anti-TB drug (any resistance) among previously treated TB patients was much higher (25.1%) (varying from 0% to 86%). The proportion of MDR-TB among previously treated TB patients ranged from 0% to 65.1%. Several countries/territories of the former Soviet Union reported >12% of all new cases as MDR-TB [22].

According to more recent data, 3.7% of new cases and 20% of previously treated cases worldwide are now estimated to have MDR-TB. Globally, there were an estimated 630,000 cases of MDR-TB among the world's 12 million prevalent cases of TB in 2011 [21]. However, only a fraction of these MDR-TB cases were actually notified while the remaining cases were only based on projections. This is reflected by the fact that the number of cases of MDR-TB notified in the 27 high MDR-TB burden countries has been increasing in recent years and reached almost 60,000 in 2011, yet the numbers only represent one in five (19%) of the TB patients estimated to have MDR-TB. The 27 high MDR-TB burden countries now account for >90% of MDR-TB cases and only four countries (India, China, Russian Federation and South Africa) account for ~60% of all MDR-TB cases. The highest proportion of MDR-TB cases are found in eastern Europe and central Asia [21, 22, 24]. The XDR-TB (defined as infection with MDR-TB strains additionally resistant to a fluoroquinolone and injectable agent such as kanamycin, amikacin or capreomycin) was detected in 84 countries. Nearly 9% of all MDR-TB cases are now projected to have XDR-TB and an estimated 25,000 cases of XDR-TB are now emerging globally every year [21]. However, the true extent of the problem of XDR-TB is not known as limited data are available from China and India that account for ~50% of all MDR-TB cases worldwide [21, 22, 25, 26]. The prevalence of XDR-TB among MDR-TB cases in some surveys in China has been reported to vary from 12.8% to 20% while a national survey found 110,000 incident cases of MDR-TB of which 8200 (7.5%) were XDR-TB [22, 25]. The study also found that most cases of MDR-TB and XDR-TB resulted from primary transmission of infection [25]. There are also other hot-spot regions in the world [27]. For instance, a recent study from Belarus showed a record prevalence of MDR-TB in 35% and 77% of newly diagnosed and previously treated TB patients, respectively [28].

Recently, several countries including India, Iran, Italy and South Africa have also reported infections with *M. tuberculosis* strains that are apparently resistant to all tested first-line and second-line drugs [29-32]. These so-called totally drug-resistant *M. tuberculosis* (TDR-TB) strains were shown to exhibit three different sub-populations including cells with very thick cell walls during exponential phase of growth which were absent from cultures of drug-susceptible and MDR *M. tuberculosis* strains [33]. However, the definition of TDR-TB is currently vague since susceptibility tests for some first-line (EMB and PZA) and many second-line drugs are poorly reproducible (ranging from

50% to 80% in their accuracy) and the number of drugs tested varies widely among reference mycobacteriology laboratories around the world [34, 35]. The WHO Expert Committee has recently concluded that defining total drug resistance in *M. tuberculosis* is challenging and controvercial and the existing category of XDR-TB already encompasses extensive drug resistance to the most active anti-TB drugs [35]. However, the rising incidence of MDR-TB and XDR-TB strains with extensive resistance to other second-line and third-line drugs has already reminded us of the dreadful situation of only 5-6 decades earlier when putting TB patients in Sanatoria was the only option for treatment. It seems that we have come around the full circle as treatment options for some patients are no better today than what was available when Robert Koch discovered *M. tuberculosis* as the causative agent of TB in humans.

The rising incidence of MDR-TB/XDR-TB is a major threat to global public health and control of TB epidemic. Since INH is the most active drug against actively dividing *M. tuberculosis* and RIF is most effective against dormant/semi-dormant persisting bacilli, effective treatment of MDR-TB is more difficult than drug-susceptible TB and often results in relapse or treatment failure [36-38]. The MDR-TB in sputum smear-positive pulmonary TB patients, if not treated properly, represents a major potential threat as these patients can transmit it further to close contacts. Incomplete/improper treatment of MDR-TB patients amplifies drug resistance in *M. tuberculosis* strains further and leads to the emergence of XDR-TB [24]. The XDR-TB is far more difficult to treat than MDR-TB even in developed countries and it is virtually an untreatable entity in developing countries [38-41].

Chapter III

Chemotherapy for TB and Evolution of Drug-Resistant TB

Streptomycin (SM) was the first TB-specific drug that was used in mid 1940s, however, therapy of TB patients with SM alone was not effective. The British Medical Research Council in 1948 observed that the mortality rates in pulmonary TB patients treated with SM or not treated at all were the same [42]. However, most patients in the treated group had actually died as a result of relapse of disease with SM-resistant strains. In late 1940s, *para*-aminosalycilic acid (PAS) was also developed and clinical studies using combination therapy with SM and PAS were more effective. The emergence of drug-resistant *M. tuberculosis* was reduced consideraly but the duration of treatment was extremely long (>2 years). In 1952, INH was added to the multidrug treatment regimen and greatly improved the efficacy of treatment, however, complete cure still required 18 to 24 months of therapy. The treatment course for pulmonary TB was reduced to 18 months in 1960 by replacing PAS by EMB. In 1967, RIF was added to the combination therapy and reduced the duration of treatment to 9 months. Reintroduction of PZA in four-drug combination chemotherapy for TB (INH, RIF, PZA and EMB or SM) reduced the duration of therapy to only six months which has remained nearly the same till today [43-45].

Successful treatment of drug-susceptible TB depends on the duration and combination of drugs being prescribed, treatment cost, patient's adherence to treatment and adverse drug reactions. The signs for successful chemotherapy is indicated by conversion of sputum from culture positive to culture-negative within 2 months and the clearing of filtrates on chest radiograph in an additional 2-4 months [43-45]. Several drug regimens are recommended for the treatment of active TB disease and depend on many factors including primary resistance to anti-TB drugs in a given country, site of infection (pulmonary or extrapulmonary), immunological status of the patient (HIV coinfection) and economic resources for treatment. Treatment of TB may also differ in low incidence, high-income industrialized countries compared to low-income high TB incidence countries.

The recommendations of the American Thoracic Society (ATS)/Center for Disease Control and Prevention (CDC)/Infectious Disease Society of America (IDSA) are based on universal availability of facilities for mycobacterial cultures, DST for first-line drugs and chest radiographs as well as availability of second-line drugs for all TB patients [44]. These recommendations are also applicable for other developed countries that have similar infrastructure facilities and countrywide low rates (<4%) of resistance to INH. Successful treatment typically involves an initial phase of two months duration which is followed by a continuation phase of four months. The preferred treatment regimen for culture-positive pulmonary TB caused by drug-susceptible *M. tuberculosis* in both HIV-coinfected and HIV-seronegative adults advocated by ATS/CDC/IDSA includes daily (56 doses) or 5 days/week (40 doses when drugs are given under directly observed therapy, DOT) therapy with INH, RIF, PZA and EMB for 8 weeks in the initial phase of treatment. This is followed by continuation phase of 4 or 7 months. The 4 months (18 weeks) continuation phase includes daily (126 doses) or 5 days/week (90 doses when drugs are given under DOT) therapy with INH and RIF [44]. However, patients with cavitation on initial chest radiograph and positive cultures at completion of 2 months of therapy receive a 7-month continuation phase with either daily (217 doses) or thrice weekly (93 doses) therapy with INH and RIF for 31 weeks. The 6-month course is also recommended for extrapulmonary TB involving any site except meninges, for which a 9-12 month regimen is recommended. Prolonging treatment is also suggested for patients with TB in a site that is slow to respond to anti-TB therapy and addition of corticosteroids is recommended for patients with tuberculous pericarditis and tuberculous meningitis [43-45].

The WHO also strongly recommends culture and DST to guide therapy, however, these facilities are seldom available as a routine in resource poor developing countries where majority of active TB cases occur [46]. Both WHO and ATS/CDC/IDSA treatment guidelines are built around directly observed therapy short-course (DOTS) strategy in which direct observation of therapy is one of five key elements and both recommend a two-phase treatment regimen in which the TB patients in the first phase are treated with at least four first-line drugs [47]. The WHO recommends treatment regimens of 6 to 8 month duration for both HIV-coinfected and HIV-seronegative patients depending on the organ involved, sputum smear status and daily therapy with all first-line drugs, at least during the intensive phase, in patients living in high HIV-prevalence settings [48]. A seven-month continuation phase with daily therapy with INH and RIF is also recommended for patients with tubercular meningitis, miliary TB or spinal TB with neurological involvement. The WHO also recommends omitting EMB from the initial phase of treatment for patients with smear-negative non-cavitary pulmonary TB or for patients infected with fully susceptible *M. tuberculosis* strain (if DST results are available) or for young children with primary TB [46, 48].

Treatment with properly implemented DOTS strategy has a cure rate of ≥95%, reduces relapse and the emergence of drug-resistant and MDR strains of *M. tuberculosis* and treatment-limiting adverse drug reactions are usually not severe [44, 45, 49]. Treatment failure is defined as positive sputum cultures after 3 months of multidrug therapy for pulmonary TB caused by drug-susceptible organisms. Treatment of HIV-TB coinfected patients is complicated by drug-drug interactions of RIF with antiretroviral agents (mainly protease and nonnucleoside reverse transcriptase inhibitors) [44]. Other rifamycins which are equally effective against *M. tuberculosis* but have fewer drug interactions with antiretroviral agents may be substituted for RIF [44]. Another problem associated with therapy in HIV-TB coinfection is a temporary exacerbation of symptoms, signs or radiographic manifestations of TB in patients on antiretroviral therapy due to immune reconstitution inflammatory syndrome [4, 50]. The drug regimens may be altered with other drug combinations that are likely to cause less problematic drug-drug interactions [51-53]. Another concern realized recently is the complexity in treatment of TB patients with other common co-morbidities such as diabetes. A recent prospective study of treatment outcome, recurrence and relapse in diabetes patients with TB showed that pulmonary TB had more severe clinical manifestations, delayed sputum conversion, and a higher probability of treatment failure, recurrence and relapse [54]. As the diabetes epidemic is growing worldwide, it may soon be necessary to add diabetes prevention and control in strategies of TB control and treatment similar to the current situation with HIV coinfection.

Prolonged multidrug therapy for TB is justified since *M. tuberculosis* grows very slowly with a relatively long generation time (~24 hours) and has increased capacity for dormancy with accompanying low metabolic activity. There are also distinct sub-populations of tubercle bacilli such as those located in pulmonary cavities, pus, solid caseous material or immune cells (e.g. macrophages), where the penetration of therapeutic agents is difficult or the pH is quite low (e.g. phagosome) that inhibits the activity of most anti-TB drugs. These features make *M. tuberculosis* a difficult organism to treat with therapeutic drugs [43-45]. Multidrug therapy for an extended period effectively eradicates three different types (actively dividing bacilli, slowly growing bacilli inside immune cells and persisting semidormant bacilli present extracellularly in solid caseous lesions) of bacterial populations [43, 45]. Actively growing extracellular bacilli present in liquefied caseous material of tuberculous lesions are efficiently killed by INH and RIF. PZA, active at pH below 6.0 is the most active drug followed by RIF on slowly growing bacilli inside immune cells such as macrophages. The persisting semidormant bacilli are mainly killed by RIF. Thus, RIF and PZA have a crucial role in achieving sterile eradication of the pathogen [43]. Treatment of pulmonary TB occurs in two stages. The first stage requires rapid elimination of actively growing extracellular bacilli in the lung to attain sputum smear-negative status (non-infectious state) to prevent further transmission of the disease. The second stage is slow as it requires complete sterilization and elimination of less actively growing, semi-dormant or dormant bacilli persisting intracellularly in various cell types [43-45].

Combination therapy with anti-TB drugs is also required to suppress the evolution of drug-resistant strains in TB patients. The *M. tuberculosis* strains develop resistance exclusively due to spontaneous mutations in existing genes that serve as drug targets and not through acquisition of new genes through plasmids from other bacteria. These strains evolve in the presence of drug-susceptible organisms in a drug-free environment and mutations conferring resistance to different anti-TB drugs are independent [55]. The bacterial load is high (10^7 to 10^9) in pulmonary TB patients with a well-developed cavity and increasing drug resistance is found among *M. tuberculosis* recovered from cavitary isolates compared with paired sputum isolates [45, 56]. The resistance conferring mutations in target genes for anti-TB drugs exist among wild-type strains at a frequency of 10^{-3} to 10^{-9}. Thus, monodrug therapy given to a patient with fully developed cavitary disease kills all susceptible bacteria but the resistant bacteria continue to grow and eventually replace the wild-type susceptible strain. Since the probability of two independent mutations conferring resistance to two anti-TB drugs in a single bacillus is much lower (10^{-12} to 10^{-15}), most TB patients do not contain any doubly-resistant strains if they have never been exposed previously to anti-TB drugs [55]. Thus, treatment with three or more effective drugs to which the strain is susceptible results in killing of all tubercle bacilli in all cell types, including those that are resistant to one drug as the latter are readily killed by other drugs in combination therapy [43, 45].

The risk of relapse increases with premature interruption of treatment due to the slow-growing nature of *M. tuberculosis* as all bacilli are not killed. Also, if an insufficient number of anti-TB drugs or inappropriate drug regimens or poor quality of anti-TB drugs are administered, there is a greater risk of emergence of drug-resistant TB due to the selection of resistant mutants [45]. The long duration of therapy also results in poor adherence to treatment by some TB patients adding further to the emergence of drug resistance. The MDR-TB strains evolve due to sequential accumulation of resistance conferring mutations in target genes to individual drugs. Thus, in TB patients infected with *M. tuberculosis* strains already resistant to INH, spontaneous mutations in some bacilli lead to further development of resistance to RIF if these patients are treated with INH and RIF alone resulting in emergence of MDR-TB strains. A similar sequence of events leads to resistance to additional drugs, resulting in the emergence of XDR-TB strains.

The emergence of MDR-TB with its associated high mortality rates, particularly among HIV-coinfected patients in the United States in early 1990s renewed interest in TB in the developed world. Drug-resistant TB and MDR-TB were recognized as a major threat to global public health and resulted in development of novel methods for rapid diagnosis and effective treatment strategies with several old and new anti-TB agents [36-38]. The drugs currently in use for the treatment of drug susceptible TB, drug-resistant TB, MDR-TB and XDR-TB are listed in Table 3.1. The anti-TB drugs are now categorized as first-line (most effective), second-line (less effective, more toxic) and third-line (reinforcing) agents based on efficacy, tolerability and data from clinical trials.

First-line (Group 1) drugs (INH, RIF, EMB and PZA) are highly efficacious, relatively less toxic and mostly bactericidal agents that facilitate oral formulations for combination therapy in both, hospital and community settings [43-45]. Wild type strains of *M. tuberculosis* are highly susceptible to these drugs.

Table 3.1. Important first-line, second-line and some third-line antitubercular agents currently in use for the treatment of drug-susceptible and drug-resistant tuberculosis

Category and drug	Chemical description	Cell process inhibited	Efficacy
Group 1: First-line oral drugs			
Isoniazid, INH	Nicotinic acid hydrazide	Mycolic acid synthesis	Bactericidal
Rifampin, RIF	Rifamycin derivative	RNA/Protein synthesis	Bactericidal
Pyrazinamide, PZA	Nicotinamide derivative	Protein synthesis	Bactericidal
Ethambutol, EMB	Ethylene diimino di-1-butanol	Lipid/cell wall synthesis	Bacteriostatic
[a]Rifabutin, RBU	Rifamycin derivative	RNA/Protein synthesis	Bactericidal
Rifapentine, RPE	Rifamycin derivative	RNA/Protein synthesis	Bactericidal
Group 2: Second-line, injectable agents			
Streptomycin, SM	Aminoglycoside	Protein synthesis	Bactericidal
Kanamycin, KAN	Aminoglycoside	Protein synthesis	Bactericidal
Amikacin, AMI	Aminoglycoside	Protein synthesis	Bactericidal
Capreomycin, CAP	Cyclic polypeptide	Protein synthesis	Bactericidal
Viomycin, VIO	Cyclic polypeptide	Protein synthesis	Bactericidal
Group 3: Second-line, fluoroquinolones			
Ciprofloxacin, CIP	Fluoroquinolone	DNA replication	Bacteriostatic
Ofloxacin, OFX	Fluoroquinolone	DNA replication	Bacteriostatic
Levofloxacin, LFX	Fluoroquinolone	DNA replication	Bactericidal[b]
Gatifloxacin, GFX	8-Methoxy-fluoroquinolone	DNA replication	Bactericidal
Moxifloxacin, MFX	8-Methoxy-fluoroquinolone	DNA replication	Bactericidal

Category and drug	Chemical description	Cell process inhibited	Efficacy
Group 4: Second-line, oral agents			
Ethionamide, ETA	Isonicotinic acid derivative	Mycolic acid synthesis	Bacteriostatic
Prothionamide, PTA	Isonicotinic acid derivative	Mycolic acid synthesis	Bacteriostatic
D-Cycloserine, CS	Serine derivative	Cell wall synthesis	Bacteriostatic
Terizidone, TZD	Serine derivative	Cell wall synthesis	Bacteriostatic
Para-amino salicylic acid, PAS	DNA replication/repair	DNA replication	Bacteriostatic
Group 5: Third-line agents			
Linezolid, LZD	Oxazolidinone derivative	Protein synthesis	Bactericidal
Amoxycillin-clavulanate, AMX-CLV	β-lactam with β-lactamase inhibitor	Cell wall synthesis	Bactericidal
Imipenem-clavulanate, IMP-CLV	Carbapenem with β-lactamase inhibitor	Cell wall synthesis	Bactericidal
Meropenem-clavulanate, MEP-CLV	Carbapenem with β-lactamase inhibitor	Cell wall synthesis	Bactericidal
Thiacetazone, TAC	Thiacetazone	Mycolic acid synthesis	Bacteriostatic
Clofazimine, CFZ	Iminophenazine derivative	Cell membrane function	Bacteriostatic

[a]Some RIF-resistant strains with specific *rpoB* mutations remain susceptible to RBU
[b]LFX is bactericidal at high doses

The use of SM, used earlier as a first-line drug, has declined in recent years and it is now regarded as a second-line agent due to the requirement of frequent patient's visits to health care facilities, much higher (>20%) rates of resistance of clinical *M. tuberculosis* isolates to SM in high TB incidence countries and the availability of more effective anti-TB drugs [5, 22, 44]. Other rifamycins (rifabutin, RBU and rifapentine, RPE), though more expensive, may be used in place of RIF in select patient populations [57, 58]. Rifabutin has fewer problematic drug interactions with antiretroviral agents and is used in HIV-coinfected patients concomitantly treated with protease and nonnucleoside reverse transcriptase inhibitors [53]. Rifapentine has much longer half-life and is being evaluated with higher or daily dosing in low-risk HIV-seronegative individuals for shortening treatment duration [58].

Second-line agents are less efficacious and more toxic than first-line anti-TB drugs and have been further divided into three different groups (Group 2 to Group 4) based on their mode of action, route of entry and mechanism of action. Group 2 includes injectable aminoglycosides (SM, kanamycin, KAN and amikacin, AMI) and cyclic polypeptides (capreomycin, CAP and viomycin, VIO) [43-45]. Cross-resistance between SM and other aminoglycosides (KAN or AMI) or cyclic polypeptides (CAP or VIO) is rarely reported. However, cross-resistance between KAN and AMI or between CAP and VIO is observed frequently and some *M. tuberculosis* strains also exhibit cross resistance between KAN/AMI and CAP/VIO [59, 60]. Flouroquinolones (FQs) (Group 3 oral/injectable agents) include ofloxacin (OFX), levofloxacin (LFX), moxifloxacin (MFX) and gatifloxacin (GFX). Higher doses of older FQs, OFX and LFX, have been safely administered and LFX at higher dose is bactericidal [61, 62]. The new-generation FQs (MFX and GFX) are bactericidal and are currently undergoing clinical trials for use as first-line agents to shorten treatment duration of drug-susceptible TB [63-66]. Group 4 includes oral agents that are mainly bacteriostatic, less efficacious, expensive and more toxic than other second-line drugs. Group 4 agents are added to therapy regimens only for the treatment of drug-resistant TB, MDR-TB and XDR-TB based on actual or projected susceptibility of *M. tuberculosis* strains, cost, and side-effect profiles. These agents include ethionamide (ETA), prothionamide (PTA), D-cycloserine (CS), terizidone (TZD), and *para*-amino salicylic acid (PAS) (Table 3.1) [44, 45, 67]. High dose INH and RBU may also be used as second-line oral agents for some patients with drug-resistant TB [67, 68].

Several other drugs have also been used recently for the treatment of patients with drug-resistant TB, MDR-TB and XDR-TB with varying degree of success. These third-line (Group 5) reinforcing agents are not recommended for routine use due to variable efficacy and serious side effects. The WHO has also issued guidelines for using these second-line and third-line drugs for the treatment of TB patients under national TB control programs of various countries [48, 69]. Group 5 drugs currently being used for the treatment of various forms of drug-resistant TB include linezolid (LZD) at full or half dose (to reduce toxicity) [70-72] amoxicillin-clavulanate (AMX-CLV), imipenem-clavulanate (IMP-CLV), meropenem-clavulanate (MEP-CLV) [70, 73, 74], thiacetazone (TAC) [70, 75] and clofazimine (CFZ) [70, 75]. CFZ has good potential to contribute to regimens in the treatment of MDR-TB while TAC is highly toxic and is contraindicated for HIV-coinfected TB patients [70]. *Mycobacterium tuberculosis* has intrinsic inducible resistance to clarithromycin due to *erm(37)* gene expression, however, its activity may be enhanced by concomitant use of sub-inhibitory concentrations of tobramycin [76, 77].

Chapter IV

Anti-TB Drugs: Mechanism of Action and Molecular Basis of Resistance

The resistance of *M. tuberculosis* to anti-TB drugs is caused almost exclusively due to spontaneous chromosomal mutations (nucleotide insertions, deletions or substitutions resulting in missense mutation or alteration or loss of RNA/protein function) occurring at a predictable rate (from $\sim 10^{-3}$ for PZA to $\sim 10^{-9}$ for RIF) in target genes that result in reduced susceptibility of the target to a specific anti-TB drug [78-80]. The current knowledge of the genes and their target regions involved in mediating resistance of *M. tuberculosis* to first-line and some other important anti-TB drugs is summarized in Table 4.1. The publicly available TB Drug Resistance Mutation Database (TBDReaMDB) (http://www.tdbreamdb.com) provides all reported mutations associated with resistance of *M. tuberculosis* to anti-TB drugs allowing comprehensive worldwide survey of resistance associated mutations and a platform for developing assays for molecular diagnosis of drug-resistant TB [81].

Isoniazid (isonicotinic acid hydrazide, INH) (minimum inhibitory concentration, MIC of 0.02-0.2 mg/L) is an important first-line drug that has the highest activity against actively dividing *M. tuberculosis* [82, 83]. The early bactericidal activity (EBA) (0-2 days) of INH at standard dose of 300 mg is 0.58 (range 0.431-0.77) [84]. INH is a pro-drug that is mainly activated by catalase-peroxidase encoded by *katG*. Activated INH mainly targets NADH-specific enoyl-acyl carrier protein (ACP) reductase (encoded by *inhA*) and β-ketoacyl ACP synthase (encoded by *kasA*) involved in mycolic acid synthesis.

Depletion of mycolic acids results in bacterial killing [82]. The molecular basis of resistance to INH is complex. Although mutations (insertions, deletions including complete gene loss and missense/nonsense point mutations) in *katG* gene that abolish the activation of INH are the primary mechanism conferring resistance of *M. tuberculosis* to INH, overproduction of InhA protein due to mutations in the regulatory region as well as specific point mutations in *inhA* structural gene also confer resistance to INH and the related drug, ethionamide (ETA) [78-83, 85]. Mutations found in *ahpC* (alkyl-hydroperoxide reductase) gene are compensatory, resulting from the loss of catalase-peroxidase activity and do not confer resistance to INH. Mutations in other genes (such as *iniBAC*, *ndh* and other genes) have a minor role in INH resistance [78-80, 86].

Despite this complexity, clinically relevant, high-level resistance to INH is mainly due to mutations within the *katG* gene while mutations in *inhA* regulatory region confer low-level of resistance to INH in most clinical *M. tuberculosis* isolates [78-80]. Mutations within the *katG* gene occur most frequently between codons 138 to 328, particularly at codon 315 (*katG315)* and their frequency varies from ~50% to 95% depending upon the ethnicity of the infected TB patient or geographical location where INH-resistant *M. tuberculosis* strain is isolated [86-90]. Mutations in the *inhA* regulatory region mostly occur at positions -15 and -8 (relative to *mabA* translational start site) and the frequency of these mutations in INH-resistant strains also varies greatly (from ~6% to 43%) [86, 90-92]. In earlier studies, no resistance conferring mutations were identified in some INH-resistant strains implying involvement of additional targets [86]. More recent studies involving extensive genomic characterization or complete genome sequencing have identified additional drug targets, however, their contribution remains small and not fully defined [93-95]. Induction of efflux pumps due to chromosomal mutations has also been shown recently as the first step in a general pathway leading to drug resistance in mycobacteria. Thus, prolonged serial exposure of *M. tuberculosis* strains to critical concentrations of isoniazid resulted in development of resistance to isoniazid that could be reduced by means of efflux pump inhibitors [96, 97]. Other novel mechanisms have also been elucidated recently showing that INH can be inactivated by some enzyme activities of *M. tuberculosis* causing drug resistance development [98, 99].

Table 4.1. Main gene targets conferring resistance to first-line and some second-line antitubercular agents used for the treatment of drug-susceptible and drug-resistant tuberculosis

Anti-TB drug[a]	Gene target	Encoded Product	Main target region	Codon/nucleotide mostly mutated	Level of resistance
RIF	*rpoB*	β-Subunit of RNA polymerase	81 bp RRDR[b]	S531, H526	High
RIF	*rpoB*	β-Subunit of RNA polymerase	N-terminal region	V146	High
INH	*katG*	Catalase/peroxidase	Entire gene	S315	High
INH/ETA	*inhA*	Enoyl-ACP reductase	Regulatory region	-15 C	Low
INH	*inhA*	Enoyl-ACP reductase	Few codons	None	Low
PZA	*pncA*	Pyrazinamidase	Many codons	None	High
PZA	*rpsA*	Ribosomal S1 Protein	C-terminal region	None	Low
EMB	*embB*	Arabinosyl transferase	Many codons	M306	Low
EMB	*embA*	Arabinosyl transferase	Many codons	None	Low
SM	*rpsL*	Ribosomal S12 Protein	Few codons	K43, K88	High
SM	*rrs*	16S rRNA	Few nucleotides	None	Low
SM	*gidB*	m7G methyltransferase	Few codons	None	Low
ETA/TAC	*ethA*	mono-oxygenase	Many codons	None	High
FQs	*gyrA*	DNA gyrase, A subunit	QRDR	A90, D94	High
FQs	*gyrB*	DNA gyrase, B subunit	Few codons	None	High
KAN/AMI	*rrs*	16S rRNA	3'-end of 16S rRNA	A1401	High
KAN	*eis*	Aminoglycoside acetyltransferase	Regulatory region	-14 C	Low

Table 4.1. (Continued)

Anti-TB drug[a]	Gene target	Encoded Product	Main target region	Codon/nucleotide mostly mutated	Level of resistance
CAP	*rrs*	16S rRNA	3'-end of 16S rRNA	A1401	Low
CAP/VIO	*tlyA*	Cytotoxin/haemolysin homologue	Several codons	None	Low
VIO	*rrs*	16S rRNA	3'-end of 16S rRNA	G1484	High
PAS	*thyA*	Thymidylate synthase	Few codons	T202	High

[a] RIF, rifampicin; INH, isoniazid; ETA, ethionamide; PZA, pyrazinamide; EMB, ethambutol; TAC, thiacetazone; FQs, fluoroquinolones (ofloxacin, levofloxacin, gatifloxacin and moxifloxacin); KAN, kanamycin; AMI, amikacin; CAP, capreomycin; VIO, viomycin; PAS, para-amino salicylic acid

[b] RRDR, rifampicin resistance determining region

Rifampicin (RIF) (MIC of 0.2-0.4 mg/L), a rifamycin derivative, together with INH, forms the backbone of short-course combination chemotherapy for active TB disease due to its excellent bactericidal activity for dormant or slowly metabolizing (persisters) *M. tuberculosis*. Other rifamycins such as RPE and RBU are also active against *M. tuberculosis* with similar MIC values. RPE has a longer half-life than RIF while RBU has fewer drug-drug interactions, and is particularly useful in HIV-coinfected TB patients [57, 100]. RIF binds to β-subunit of RNA polymerase (encoded by *rpoB*) and inhibits RNA transcription and thus, protein synthesis in *M. tuberculosis* [78-80, 101]. The EBA (0-2 days) of RIF at standard dose of 600 mg is 0.21 (range 0.174-0.299) [84]. Mutations in *rpoB* gene confer RIF resistance by affecting drug binding. Monoresistance to RIF is rare except in patients coinfected with HIV or with some other underlying disease [102-105]. Since nearly 85-90% of RIF-resistant *M. tuberculosis* isolates are also resistant to INH, resistance to RIF is regarded as a surrogate marker for MDR-TB [37, 78-80].

Global molecular epidemiological studies have shown that 90-95% of RIF-resistant *M. tuberculosis* isolates contain missense mutations or small insertions/deletions located usually within an 81-bp hot-spot region (rifampicin resistance determining region, RRDR) spanning *rpoB* codons 507-533 (*Escherichia coli* numbering system) [101, 106-113]. Mutations occur most commonly at codons 531, 526 or 516 with S531L, H526Y, H526D and D516V mutations occurring in 70-95% of RIF-resistant *M. tuberculosis* isolates in most countries/settings. Resistance in 5%-10% of RIF-resistant isolates is due to mutations in N-terminal (codon V146) or cluster II regions of *rpoB* gene or due to mutations in other genes [114-118]. Induction of efflux pumps may also lead to multidrug resistance in *M. tuberculosis* and this resistance can be reduced by means of efflux pumps inhibitors [97]. Specific mutations in RRDR, N-terminal and cluster II regions also show variations depending upon the ethnicity of TB patient and/or the geographical location where *M. tuberculosis* strain is isolated [37, 106-113, 119].

There is also a correlation between substitutions at specific amino acids in the *rpoB* gene and MIC of RIF for *M. tuberculosis*. High-level of RIF resistance is associated with missense mutations in codons 146, 526 and 531 while substitutions at codons 511, 518 and 522 cause low-level of RIF resistance [78-80, 106, 112, 120]. There is also a relationship between specific *rpoB* mutations and cross-resistance of *M. tuberculosis* isolates to other rifamycins (RPE and RBU). While cross-resistance to RIF and RPE is very common, nearly 12-20% RIF-resistant strains, including some MDR-TB strains, remain susceptible to RBU [121-124]. Thus, RBU may be used as an alternative second-line drug for the treatment of some patients infected with RIF-resistant strains carrying specific *rpoB* mutations. Other rifamycin derivatives have also been synthesized recently that show more powerful *in vitro* activities than RIF or RBU against wild-type and RIF-resistant, including multidrug-resistant, *M. tuberculosis* strains [125, 126].

Since RIF targets catalytic subunit of RNA polymerase (*rpoB*), an enzyme required for gene expression leading to synthesis of RNA and proteins, the fitness of RIF-resistant *M. tuberculosis* strains has been the subject of much speculation until recently. Most RIF-resistant *M. tuberculosis* strains selected *in vitro* have reduced fitness while RIF-resistant clinical *M. tuberculosis* isolates with multiple mutations in the *rpoB* gene are transmitted to other hosts, suggesting a role of secondary compensatory mutations for improving the fitness of a primary mutation in the *rpoB* gene. Recent studies based on complete genome sequencing of susceptible, RIF-resistant and multidrug-resistant *M. tuberculosis* strains have shown that compensatory mutations are indeed found in other RNA polymerase (*rpoA, rpoC*) genes resulting in high competitive fitness of RIF-resistant mutants. These mutations were absent in RIF-susceptible clinical *M. tuberculosis* strains [95, 127].

Pyrazinamide (PZA), a pro-drug, is a structural analog of nicotinamide and is highly effective against semidormant bacilli residing in acidic environment (like inside phagosome in macrophages) [43]. PZA is activated by pyrazinamidase encoded by *pncA* gene to pyrazinoic acid which, by lowering intracellular pH, inactivates a vital step in fatty acid synthesis in *M. tuberculosis* [78-80, 128]. The activity of PZA is highly specific against *M. tuberculosis,* other mycobacteria are intrinsically resistant to PZA due to lack of an efficient drug-activating enzyme (pyrazinamidase). Ribosomal protein S1 encoded by *rpsA* that is involved in protein translation and ribosome-sparing process of translation, an activity essential for non-replicating tubercle bacilli has also been identified recently as another cellular target of pyrazinoic acid in *M. tuberculosis* [129]. These findings have confirmed the sterilizing role of PZA by eradicating persisting organisms during the course of chemotherapy. Being a pro-drug, most PZA-resistant *M. tuberculosis* strains, similar to INH, also contain mutations in *pncA*, the gene encoding pyrazinamidase that activates the pro-drug. Some PZA-resistant *M. tuberculosis* strains also contain mutations in *rpsA* [128-133]. Some PZA resistant *M. tuberculosis* isolates contain wild-type *pncA* and *rpsA* genes suggesting the existence of other PZA resistance conferring mechanism(s) in *M. tuberculosis* [129-133].

Ethambutol (EMB), an ethylene diamine derivative, with an MIC value of 0.5-2.0 mg/L, is now used as the fourth drug in oral formulations of combination therapy for TB recommended by WHO and ATS/CDC/IDSA in place of SM since worldwide prevalence of resistance of *M. tuberculosis* strains to EMB is much lower compared to SM and use of SM also requires frequent patient's visits to the health care facilities [5, 22, 44]. Also, the EBA (0-2 days) at the recommended doses of EMB (15 mg/kg) and SM (20 mg/kg) are nearly same [84]. EMB inhibits synthesis and polymerization of cell wall arabinan, which is required for important cell wall components such as arabinogalactan and lipoarabinomannan. Inhibition of arabinan synthesis leads to accumulation of free mycolic acids resulting in incomplete cell wall assembly and cell death. The drug mainly interacts with membrane associated arabinosyltransferases encoded by three contiguous genes (*embCAB* operon) as an arabinose analogue [134]. Other targets for EMB include proteins encoded by isoniazid-inducible genes particularly *iniA*, acyl carrier proteins and regulatory proteins modulating the expression of acyl carrier proteins [135].

The mechanism of action and the molecular genetic basis of resistance to EMB are complex and are not completely defined. Resistance conferring mutations in three *emb* genes have been identified in clinical *M. tuberculosis* strains and mutations in *embB* occur more frequently, particularly at *embB* codon 306 (*embB306)*, *embB406* and *embB497* [134-136]. Mutations at *embB306* have also been reported in some EMB-susceptible *M. tuberculosis* isolates, particularly strains resistant to several other first-line anti-TB drugs and MDR-TB strains, likely due to the faulty phenotypic DST of *M. tuberculosis* for slow-acting EMB [137-139]. Recent studies have shown that *embB306* mutations in *M. tuberculosis* isolates only cause slight increase in MIC values which is sometimes missed by inconsistent phenotypic DST methods [140-142]. Similar to the frequency of mutations conferring resistance to INH and RIF, the frequency of *embB306* mutations also varies considerably (25% to 70%) in EMB-resistant clinical *M. tuberculosis* strains isolated from different geographical locations [134-136, 143, 144]. Since some EMB-resistant *M. tuberculosis* strains do not contain a resistance conferring mutation in all genes currently implicated in EMB resistance, other mechanisms exist and need to be worked out, possibly by complete genome sequencing of selected EMB-resistant *M. tuberculosis* strains [93, 95, 135].

Streptomycin (SM) (MIC of 0.5-2 mg/L) is nearly as effective as EMB, however, several factors (as stated above) have discouraged its widespread use in recent years. According to the recommendations of ATS/CDC/IDSA, SM and EMB are not considered as interchangeable unless the cultured *M. tuberculosis* isolate from the TB patient is known to be susceptible to SM or if the TB patient is from an ethnic group/geographical location where SM resistance is highly unlikely [44]. The SM may be used for treating patients with failing therapy or MDR-TB only if the infecting *M. tuberculosis* strain is susceptible to SM [145]. The bactericidal action of SM is due to its binding to the small subunit of ribosomes that causes faulty protein synthesis due to misreading of mRNA during translation. The drug specifically binds to the 12S ribosomal protein, RpsL and 16S rRNA (*rrs*) within the 30S (small) subunit of the ribosomes and inhibits protein synthesis [78-80]. Since *M. tuberculosis* genome contains a single copy of *rrs* gene, alteration in *rrs* gene can also potentially cause SM resistance [2]. Indeed, nearly 30% of SM-resistant clinical *M. tuberculosis* isolates contain mutations in the *rrs* gene [146]. However, mutations in *rrs* gene cause only low-level of resistance to SM. High-level resistance to SM in *M. tuberculosis* isolates usually involves missense mutations in *rpsL*, particularly at *rpsL* codon 43 (*rpsL43*) and *rpsL88* [146-148]. Another target recently identified that also confers low-level resistance to SM in *M. tuberculosis* is *gidB* gene, encoding 7-methylguanosine (m7G) methyltransferase that is specific for 16S rRNA [148]. The involvement of efflux pumps has also been shown recently in mediating resistance of *M. tuberculosis* to SM and mutations in *gidB* and an efflux pump were recently shown to act synergistically to confer low-level of resistance to SM [149].

Other injectable aminoglycosides, kanamycin (KAN) and amikacin (AMI) with MIC values of 0.5-2 mg/L also inhibit protein synthesis in *M. tuberculosis* and are active against actively dividing bacteria [43-45, 78-80]. The EBA (0-2 days) of standard dose of KAN/AMI for *M. tuberculosis* is also nearly same as of SM [84]. Although cross-resistance between KAN and AMI has been reported, they may be used for SM-resistant *M. tuberculosis* strains as second-line injectable agents since cross-resistance between SM and KAN/AMI is rarely reported [78-80, 150]. Due to lower resistance rates to these drugs among clinical *M. tuberculosis* isolates as compared to SM, excellent bactericidal activity and availability of limited drug options, both KAN and AMI are now widely used for the treatment of MDR-TB [36-38, 44]. Cyclic polypeptides, capreomycin (CAP) and viomycin (VIO) with similar MIC values (1-4 mg/L) also inhibit protein synthesis, are bactericidal against actively dividing *M. tuberculosis* and are also used as alternative second-line injectable drugs for the treatment of MDR-TB [36-38, 44].

Resistance to KAN and AMI in *M. tuberculosis* is mainly associated with mutations in the 3'-end of *rrs* gene [59, 60]. Mutations in the 3'-end of *rrs* gene and *tlyA*, encoding rRNA methyltransferase confer resistance to CAP and/or VIO [59, 60, 151, 152]. The *M. tuberculosis* strains with mutations in the *tlyA* gene remain susceptible to KAN and AMI. Cross-resistance between KAN and AMI or between KAN and CAP or VIO is observed at highly variable patterns and strains resistant to KAN, AMI and CAP but susceptible to VIO have been described [59, 150, 153, 154]. Mutation A1401G in the *rrs* gene causes high-level of resistance to KAN and AMI but usually causes low-level resistance to CAP in *M. tuberculosis*. Mutations C1402T and G1484T in the *rrs* gene have also been detected in some *M. tuberculosis* strains resistant to KAN, AMI and/or CAP, however, other studies did not detect these mutations in drug-resistant strains [60, 153]. The contribution of *tlyA* mutations in conferring resistance to CAP is minor [60, 153]. Another mechanism conferring low-level resistance to KAN *in M. tuberculosis* involves upregulation (due to promoter mutations) of aminoglycoside acetyltransferase encoded by *eis* gene which inactivates the drug [155]. Interestingly, some strains resistant to KAN, AMI and CAP but susceptible to SM have also been described recently indicating that SM may also be useful in the treatment of some XDR *M. tuberculosis* strains [150].

Fluoroquinolones (FQs) are oral, broad-spectrum bactericidal antimicrobial agents recently introduced for the treatment of TB [62, 156, 157]. The older FQs, such as ciprofloxacin (CIP, MIC of 0.25-2 mg/L) and ofloxacin (OFX, MIC of 0.25-2 mg/L) are safer drugs but are only moderately active against *M. tuberculosis* strains. Higher doses of CIP (1500 mg) and OFX (800 mg) have also been used safely but are bacteriostatic for tubercle bacilli. The EBA (0-2 days) for even high dose CIP and OFX are modest and have been reported as 0.21 and 0.32-0.38, respectively [62, 84]. The CIP is no longer used due to its poor activity while OFX, due to its lower cost, is still being used in some developing countries for the treatment of MDR-TB. New generation FQs such as levofloxacin (LFX, MIC of 0.25-2 mg/L), moxifloxacin (MFX, MIC of 0.125-0.5 mg/L) and gatifloxacin (GFX, MIC of 0.062-0.5 mg/L) are more potent anti-TB agents. LFX at high dose (1000 mg) and GFX and MFX at regular dose (400 mg each) exhibit EBA (0-2 days) values of 0.45, 0.35 and 0.33-0.53 for LFX, GFX and MFX, respectively, which are close to that of INH [61, 84]. The potent EBA of MFX and GFX, against *M. tuberculosis* and once daily oral dosing make these drugs highly desirable agents for combination therapy of fully susceptible pulmonary TB. These drugs have been evaluated for shortening the treatment duration of fully susceptible pulmonary TB with encouraging results and further evaluations are currently underway [63-66]. FQs (MFX and GFX as well as high dose OFX and LFX are also useful as second-line agents for the treatment of drug-resistant TB, MDR-TB and XDR-TB as well as for TB patients who are intolerant to some of the first-line drugs [37, 44, 62, 156, 157].

Like other bacteria, the cellular target of FQs in *M. tuberculosis* is also DNA gyrase (a type II topoisomerase) consisting of two A and two B subunits encoded by *gyrA* and *gyrB* genes, respectively. Inhibition of DNA gyrase activity by FQs results in inhibition of DNA replication, transcription and repair, causing cell death [156]. Clinical *M. tuberculosis* isolates with wild-type *gyrA* and *gyrB* gene sequences are highly susceptible to FQs while chromosomal mutations in clinical *M. tuberculosis* strains in *gyrA* and *gyrB* genes confer resistance to FQs [62, 156]. Missense mutations in small regions of *gyrA* and *gyrB* genes, called quinolone resistance-determining region (QRDR) confer resistance to FQs in clinical *M. tuberculosis* isolates [62, 156, 158]. In some *M. tuberculosis* strains, changes in the drug efflux pump systems may also result in low-level resistance to FQs [159]. Mutations in *gyrA* gene occur more frequently at codon 90 or 94 while mutations in few codons of the *gyrB* gene occur in a small minority of clinical FQ-resistant *M. tuberculosis* strains [160-163]. Cross-resistance between different FQs is generally assumed since all FQs share the same drug targets (*gyrA* and *gyrB*), however, it is not 100%. There are some reports that indicate that certain mutations in *gyrA* and *gyrB* confer FQ resistance but the level and pattern of resistance varies among the different mutations. Thus, not all OFX-resistant strains are resistant to MFX. Similarly, some *M. tuberculosis* strains resistant to MFX remain susceptible to OFX [158, 162-165]. These findings have important implications for the use of FQs in the treatment of patients infected with XDR-TB strains.

Ethionamide (2-ethylisonicotinamide, ETA) is a structural analog of INH and, with an MIC of 2.5-10.0 mg/L, is frequently used as an efficacious second-line drug for the treatment of MDR-TB and XDR-TB [36, 39, 44]. ETA is also a pro-drug and like INH, targets *inhA*, involved in mycolic acid biosynthesis [85]. Cross-resistance between INH and ETA has long been known. Low-level INH-resistant *M. tuberculosis* strains frequently display ETA resistance while high-level INH-resistant strains typically due to *katG* mutations remain ETA susceptible [78-80]. Prothionamide (PTA), another pro-drug, shares the same structure and its activity is also almost identical to ETA. Both, ETA and PTA are activated to their active form (4-ethyl-4-amidopyridine) in a two-step reaction catalyzed by a monooxygenase (encoded by *ethA*) yielding etionamide-NAD adduct [166, 167]. The *ethA* also activates other thioamide drugs such as thiacetazone (TAC) [168]. Similar to other pro-drugs, INH and PZA, majority of ETA-resistant *M. tuberculosis* strains contain mutations in *ethA* that abolish activation of pro-drug [78, 169]. The *ethA* mutations also cause cross-resistance to other thioamides such as TAC. As the main cellular target of activated ETA is *inhA*, mutations in *inhA* (regulatory region as well as the structural gene) confer resistance to both, ETA and INH [168, 169]. The *mshA* gene encoding a glycosyltransferase involved in mycothiol biosynthesis is another possible target of ETA [170]. Another mechanism conferring resistance to ETA involves inactivation of the drug by NADH pyrophosphatase encoded by *nudC* gene [98].

The molecular mechanisms conferring resistance to some other second-line and third-line anti-TB drugs have also been elucidated recently. In addition to *ethA*, mutations in β-hydroxyacyl ACP dehydratase complex, an essential type 2 fatty acid synthase, result in high-level of resistance to TAC in *M. tuberculosis* [171]. D-cycloserine, an analog of D-alanine inhibits the synthesis of peptidoglycan by blocking the action of D-alanine:D-alanine ligase and overproduction of D-alanine recemase and D-alanine:D-alanine ligase confers resistance to D-cycloserine in mycobacteria [172]. D-cycloserine is taken up in *M. tuberculosis* by a transporter protein encoded by *cycA* gene. A single point mutation in *cycA* gene disrupts the uptake of D-cycloserine and confers resistance to this drug in *M. tuberculosis,* however, partial contribution of this impairment suggests the involvement of additional genetic loci in this resistance phenotype [173]. Two thymidylate synthase enzymes (encoded by *thyA* and *thyX*) catalyse the biosynthesis of deoxythymidine monophosphate (TMP) in *M. tuberculosis* and thus are important for DNA replication and repair. The cellular target of PAS in *M. tuberculosis* is thymidylate synthase enzyme encoded by *thyA*. Deletion or point mutations in *thyA* confer PAS resistance in *M. tuberculosis* while *thyX* is an essential gene suggesting its role in other functions besides TMP synthesis [174, 175]. Linezolid (LZD) inhibits protein synthesis by binding to the large (50S) subunit and mutations in *rrl* encoding 23S rRNA confer resistance to linezolid [176]. More recently, mutations in *rplC* encoding the ribosomal L3 protein have also been identified as another target in LZD-resistant *M. tuberculosis* strains [177].

Chapter V

Diagnosis of Active TB Disease

The diagnosis of active disease (including pulmonary as well as extrapulmonary TB) is usually based on clinical suspicion, chest radiographs and laboratory diagnosis by smear microscopic examination for acid-fast bacilli (AFB), growth of *M. tuberculosis* by solid or liquid culture and, more recently, by detection of *M. tuberculosis* nucleic acid in clinical specimens [38, 178-180]. The gold standard for the diagnosis of active disease is culture of *M. tuberculosis* on solid or liquid media [178-180]. Culture also allows DST against first-line and selected second-line drugs for detection of MDR-TB and XDR-TB. Some molecular tests developed recently for the diagnosis of active TB disease directly in clinical specimens also detect resistance of *M. tuberculosis* to RIF [178-181]. Since ~85-90% of RIF-resistant *M. tuberculosis* isolates are also resistant to INH (except in some select patient populations such as HIV-coinfected individuals), detection of RIF resistance also identifies majority of MDR-TB strains [27, 78-80].

The microscopic examination of smears for AFB is routinely used to diagnose TB in resource-limited settings. However, the sensitivity of smear microscopy by Ziehl-Neelsen staining for expectorated sputum is only 34-80% of positive cultures. The sensitivity of *M. tuberculosis* detection has improved recently by using auramine O fluorochrome and light emitting diode technology [178]. The sensitivity of smear examination for extrapulmonary samples is even lower, the test does not differentiate TB from infections caused by non-tuberculous mycobacteria (NTM) and DST is not feasible. Also, microscopy is often negative in HIV-coinfected pulmonary TB patients due to paucibacillary load [178, 182].

The culture of *M. tuberculosis* is the gold standard for TB diagnosis, especially in smear-negative specimens and allows species-specific identification, DST to guide therapy and fingerprinting of *M. tuberculosis* strains during epidemics to trace the source of infection [44, 178-180]. Culture on conventional solid (Lowenstein-Jensen) medium is time-consuming requiring at least 4-6 weeks for detectable growth and species-specific identification requires a further 2-3 weeks [23, 183]. The liquid (like Middlebrook 7H9) media have reduced the turn-around time considerably for culture positivity. Semi-automated and more recently fully automated liquid culture systems (such as BACTEC mycobacteria growth indicator tube, MGIT 960 culture system) have allowed recovery of mycobacteria from a variety of clinical specimens within 14 days, however, additional time and labor is needed for identification of *M. tuberculosis* [23, 184]. Due to high cost of automated liquid culture systems, other rapid liquid culture-based methods have also been developed recently for resource-limited settings. All culture-based systems require biosafety laboratory category 3 facilities and training of personnel to avoid exposure to *M. tuberculosis*.

The liquid cultures of automated systems can be directly used for rapid identification of *M. tuberculosis* by using molecular methods [179, 183]. The commercial Accuprobe assay can identify *M. tuberculosis* and five common NTM species (*M. avium, M. intracellulare, M. avium* complex, *M. kansasii,* and *M. gordonae*) in ~2 hours from culture-positive tubes [185]. Two commercial reverse hybridization-based line probe assays (INNO-LiPA MYCOBACTERIA v2 and Genotype *Mycobacterium* assay) have been developed for identification of *M. tuberculosis* and several NTM species, both in cultured isolates and clinical specimens [186-188]. PCR sequencing of fragments of conserved genes such as 16S rRNA, 16S-23S internal transcribed spacer region, *rpoB*, 65-kilodalton heat shock protein (*hsp65*) and *secA1* have also been used for identification of *M. tuberculosis* and NTM species [179, 183, 189]. Matrix-assisted laser desorption/ionization-time of flight mass spectrometry (MALDI-TOF MS) has also been used for rapid identification of *Mycobacterium* spp. from fresh liquid and solid cultures [190, 191]. Although rapid, these methods are expensive, technically demanding and thus not suitable for most of the poor developing countries where majority of active TB disease cases occur.

More recently, other simple and rapid immunological methods have also been developed. These include commercially available oligochromatographic test (Speed-Oligo Mycobacteria) for rapid detection of *M. tuberculosis* complex and several NTM species in culture-positive samples and two immunochromatographic assays detecting the presence of MPT64 antigen that is specifically secreted by *M. tuberculosis* in culture medium [192-194]. The immunochromatographic assays are simple, rapid (requiring <1 hour) and relatively inexpensive than molecular probes for definitive laboratory diagnosis of TB and are suitable for countries where majority of mycobacterial infections are caused by *M. tuberculosis*.

Molecular methods, typically involving PCR/real-time PCR, have also been developed recently for the diagnosis of active TB disease directly in clinical specimens [178-180, 189]. These assays are recommended as additional evidence of infection and for identification of *M. tuberculosis* in sputum smear-positive specimens. The in-house PCR and real-time PCR assays vary greatly in amplification target and detection platforms and the sensitivity and reliability of these tests also vary considerably. Commercially available tests perform better and some are also approved by Food and Drug Administration (FDA) of the United States of America and WHO for routine diagnosis of TB. The tests currently available commercially include Cobas TaqMan MTB test [195, 196], Amplified Mycobacterium Tuberculosis Direct (AMTD) test [197], BDProbeTec ET *Mycobacterium tuberculosis* complex direct detection assay [198] and the GeneXpert MTB/RIF (Xpert MTB/RIF) assay [181, 195-197]. These tests are approved mainly for respiratory specimens particularly, smear-positive samples as their sensitivity is usually lower for smear-negative samples. Pooled sensitivity of these tests for smear-positive and smear-negative respiratory samples is ~95% and ~70%, respectively, while their performance in extra-pulmonary specimens (particularly smear-negative samples) is usually much lower [179, 180].

The launch of Xpert MTB/RIF assay has provided a point of care test for the diagnosis of active TB disease. This single cartridge-based fully automated, real-time PCR amplification and detection system equipped with an internal control detects *M. tuberculosis* and its resistance to RIF (targeting the RRDR of the *rpoB* gene) directly in clinical samples with little processing and hands-on-time producing results in ~2 hours [181, 199]. The rapidity, simplicity and closed reaction chamber of Xpert MTB/RIF assay is less prone to contamination making it a good TB diagnostic test for routine use in both, developed and developing countries. The simultaneous detection of RIF resistance is an added advantage for countries with a high incidence of MDR-TB since ~85-90% of RIF-resistant strains are also resistant to INH [78-80]. Although originally intended for respiratory specimens, it has also performed well for a variety of non-respiratory samples [200-203]. The assay detected 98%-100% of smear-positive and 57%-83% smear-negative pulmonary disease among prospectively studied TB suspects. However, the sensitivity of 53% to 95% has been reported for extrapulmonary specimens due to variations in the range of samples and their smear status [204].

The WHO has strongly encouraged the use of Xpert MTB/RIF assay wherever possible, particularly among HIV-coinfected individuals, to control the TB epidemic and for proper management of MDR-TB [6, 21]. Following the endorsement by WHO in December 2010, the roll out of Xpert MTB/RIF assay has been truly impressive even in developing countries. Between its endorsement and the end of June 2012, 1.1 million tests had been purchased by 67 low- and middle-income countries with South Africa leading the group of countries that have adopted this rapid diagnostic test for TB. The cost of the test was subsequently reduced in August 2012 (from US $16.86 to US $ 9.98, a 41% price reduction) for wider application of this rapid test in low- and middle-income countries where majority of active TB disease cases occur every year [21]. This is indicated by the sharp increase in the number of instruments and test cartridges that have been sold subsequently. The TBXpert project is being executed and monitored by the WHO Stop TB Department and the Stop TB Partnership secretariat. According to WHO data, a total of 1,123 GeneExpert instruments (comprising 6,181 modules) and 2,315,380 Xpert MTB/RIF cartridges had been procured in the public sector alone in 83 of the 145 countries eligible for concessional pricing, as of March 31, 2013 (http://who.int/tb/laboratory/mtbrifrollout/en/). There are, however, some reports of detection of false-positive cases of RIF resistance with Xpert MTB/RIF assay, particularly in settings with low RIF resistance prevalence [205, 206]. The application of Xpert MTB/RIF assay for screening patients before antiretroviral therapy (ART) in South Africa has also resulted in much better case detection rates for TB [207]. The data suggest that screening of all patients prior to ART in high HIV-TB coinfection settings may prove to be cost effective.

Chapter VI

Diagnosis of Drug-Resistant TB, MDR-TB and XDR-TB

Rapid diagnosis of active disease is not sufficient for proper management of TB patients due to the problem of drug-resistant TB, MDR-TB and more recently, XDR-TB. Rapid detection of drug resistant *M. tuberculosis* is also essential to ensure effective treatment of TB patients which will limit the development of additional resistance to anti-TB drugs. Both, WHO and CDC advocate DST of culture isolates to first-line and second-line drugs. Phenotypic DST methods typically require solid or liquid culture while molecular tests developed recently may be applied directly on clinical specimens or *M. tuberculosis* cultures. Some molecular tests developed recently for the diagnosis of active disease (Xpert MTB/RIF) also simultaneously detect resistance to RIF and majority of MDR-TB strains [181, 199, 204]. Some of the currently available and more commonly used conventional (phenotypic) and molecular (genotypic) methods for DST of *M. tuberculosis* isolates are listed in Table 6.1 and are described below.

6A. Conventional Diagnosis of Drug-Resistant TB, MDR-TB and XDR-TB

Conventional DST is based on phenotypic detection of *M. tuberculosis* growth in the presence of antibiotic by one of three (absolute concentration, resistance ratio or proportion method) methods on solid (Lowenstein-Jensen) medium [208]. The absolute concentration method uses a standard inoculum of the test strain grown with a two-fold dilution of drug-containing and drug-free media. The resistance of an *M. tuberculosis* strain is determined as MIC, which is defined as the lowest concentration of a certain drug that nearly completely inhibits the growth of tubercle bacilli. The resistance ratio method compares the MIC of a test strain with that of standard strain, *M. tuberculosis* $H_{37}Rv$. Resistance ratio corresponds to the MIC of test strain divided by the MIC of the drug susceptible reference (*M. tuberculosis* $H_{37}Rv$) strain tested at the same time. The proportion method gives the precise proportion of resistant bacilli in a sample to a certain drug. A set of 100 fold dilutions of *M. tuberculosis* culture suspension is inoculated into drug containing and drug free (control) media. The ratio of number of colonies growing on drug containing versus control medium indicates the proportion of drug-resistant bacilli present in the culture. A cut-off value (critical proportion) defines whether the isolate is drug-susceptible or drug-resistant. Susceptibility to first-line drugs is reliable on solid medium while there is some controversy regarding standardization of DST for second-line and other anti-TB drugs. However, these methods are slow, requiring 2-4 weeks to report the results from the primary culture. The WHO favors DST for second-line drugs by automated liquid culture systems [209].

The broth-based nonradioactive, fully automated Bactec MGIT 960 TB liquid culture system has recently replaced the semiautomated, radiometric BACTEC 460 TB system regarded earlier as the gold standard for DST of *M. tuberculosis* to both first- and second-line anti-TB drugs [208-210]. Other automated liquid culture systems used for DST of *M. tuberculosis* include ESP culture system II, MB/BACT system and VersaTREK system [208, 211]. Of these, Bactec MGIT 960 TB system, reporting results within 5-8 days from a primary culture, is considered equivalent to BACTEC 460 TB system [208, 210]. The main disadvantages of automated liquid culture systems include high cost, need for an uninterrupted supply of consumables and indirect DST of *M. tuberculosis*. Recently, a multicenter study successfully carried out DST with Bactec MGIT 960 system directly from processed smear-positive specimens (direct DST) for INH and RIF to reliably detect MDR-TB cases within 8-10 days [212]. Although MGIT 960 system may be used directly on sputum samples, additional time and labor is needed for identification of *M. tuberculosis*. As automated liquid culture systems are too expensive for most of the developing countries, efforts have been made to develop simple, inexpensive non-commercial alternative phenotypic methods for resource-poor settings for the diagnosis and DST of *M. tuberculosis* [213-216]. These include microscopic observation drug susceptibility (MODS) test, thin layer agar (TLA) method, nitrate reducatse (NR) assay, the colorimetric redox indicator (CRI) methods and phage-based assays. These methods utilize inexpensive laboratory materials, limited staff training is required and most can be set up directly on clinical specimens. Of these MODS, NR and CRI assays have been endorsed by WHO [209].

The liquid media-based MODS test is a low-cost alternative for detection and DST of *M. tuberculosis* in sputum specimens for first-line drugs and results are available within a median of 7-9 days [217, 218]. The MODS test uses Middlebrook 7H9 broth containing anti-TB drugs in 24-well plates, sputum is directly inoculated and cording growth is detected as strings and tangles of *M. tuberculosis* using an inverted light microscope. A sample is considered as susceptible if growth is observed in the drug-free control wells but not in drug-containing wells and resistant if growth is observed in both control and drug-containing wells. The MODS assay has been extensively evaluated and exhibits nearly perfect agreement ($\geq$95%) with conventional DST for INH, RIF and MDR-TB [218-221]. The test has also performed well with sputum and other sample types as well as with culture isolates in several poor and developing countries and is among the most cost-effective methods that permits testing of large number of samples similar to automated culture systems [179, 216].

The TLA is another inexpensive test that only requires an incubator and light microscope. Similar to MODS test, TLA method also employs initial identification of tubercle bacilli based on cording morphology that is observed microscopically and DST results are usually available within 10-12 days [216, 218].

The method has been evaluated on primary specimens against conventional solid and liquid culture methods with good results for the detection of MDR-TB/XDR-TB in cultures [218, 222-224]. Major limitations of MODS and TLA tests include indirect identification of *M. tuberculosis* and the requirement for frequent microscopic observations [216]. However, unlike MODS test, TLA method has not yet been endorsed by WHO due to insufficient evidence of its performance. Further studies using primary clinical specimens are currently underway.

Table 6.1. Phenotypic and genotypic methods currently available for the detection of resistance of *M. tuberculosis* to first-line, second-line and third-line anti-TB drugs

Available methods for drug susceptibility testing	Susceptibility testing for detection of			Detection in sputum	Turn around time, day(s)
	Drug-resistant TB[a]	MDR-TB	XDR-TB		
Phenotypic tests					
Lowenstein-Jensen solid culture	FLDs, SLDs, TLDs	Yes	Yes	No	14-28
Indirect Bactec MGIT 960 culture	FLDs, SLDs, TLDs	Yes	Yes	No	5 to 8
Direct Bactec MGIT 960 culture	INH, RIF	Yes	No	Yes	8 to 10
MODS assay	INH, RIF, EMB, SM	Yes	No	Yes	7 to 9
Thin layer agar assay	FLDs, SLDs	Yes	Yes	Yes	10 to 12
Nitrate reductase assay	FLDs, SLDs	Yes	Yes	Yes	7 to 10
Colorimetric redox indicator assays	FLDs, SLDs	Yes	Yes	Yes	8 to 10
Luciferase reporter phage assays	INH, RIF	Yes	No	No	2 to 4
Genotypic tests					
GeneXpert MTB/RIF	RIF	Possible[b]	No	Yes	2 hours
Real-time PCR assays	FLDs	Yes	No	Yes	1 to 2
Real-time PCR with HRMC analysis[c]	FLDs, SLDs, TLDs	Yes	Yes	Yes	1 to 2
PCR-DNA sequencing/pyrosequencing	FLDs, SLDs, TLDs	Yes	Yes	Yes	1 to 2
INNO-LiPA Rif. TB line probe assay	RIF	Possible[b]	No	Yes	1 to 2
GenoType MTBDR*plus* line probe assay	INH, RIF	Yes	No	Yes	1 to 2
GenoType MTBDR*sl* line probe assay	EMB, FQs, KAN/AMI/CAP	No	Yes[d]	Yes	1 to 2

[a]Tuberculosis caused by M. tuberculosis strain resistant to indicated drugs; FLDs, first-line drugs; SLDs, second-line drugs; TLDs, third-line drugs; RIF, rifampicin; EMB, ethambutol; FQs, fluoroquinolones; KAN, kanamycin; AMI, amikacin; CAP, capreomycin

[b]Since 85-90% RIF-resistant strains are additionally resistant to isoniazid, detection of RIF resistance by this assay also detects majority of MDR-TB strains

[c]HRMC, high-resolution melting curve

[d]Detection of XDR-TB is possible when this test is combined with GenoType MTBDRplus assay

The NR assay depends on the ability of viable *M. tuberculosis* to reduce nitrate to nitrite. The production of nitrite is detected by adding other specific reagents in the culture medium which, produce a colored reaction and the results of DST are usually available within 7-10 days of incubation [179, 213, 216]. Drug-resistant *M. tuberculosis* strains reduce nitrate producing pink-red color, while susceptible strains, due to loss of viability in the presence of anti-TB drug, do not do so as their growth is inhibited by the antibiotic [213]. The NR assay has been extensively evaluated for the detection of resistance to first-line and second-line drugs and MDR-TB/XDR-TB with very high sensitivity ($\geq$95%) compared with conventional DST by proportion method on LJ medium [221, 224-226]. The NR assay, similar to MODS test, is also among the most cost-effective methods that permit simultaneous testing of a large number of samples [216]. However, unlike MODS test where cording growth of *M. tuberculosis* is used for its identification, the NR assay only detects bacterial growth and thus may yield false-positive results due to growth of other organisms. Some indeterminate results may also be obtained and the test is unable to detect rare nitrate reductase-negative *M. tuberculosis* [216].

The CRI methods are another alternative for detecting drug-resistant *M. tuberculosis* strains in resource-poor settings. They are based on reduction of redox indicators such as tetrazolium salts and resazurin, which are added to culture medium in the presence of different anti-TB drugs during *in vitro* growth of *M. tuberculosis*. The results are usually available within 8-10 days [180, 214, 216]. Resistance is detected by a change in color of the indicator, which is directly proportional to the number of viable *M. tuberculosis*. The tetrazolium salt-based assays utilize yellow colored 3-(4,5-dimethylthiazol-2-yl)-2,5-diphenyl tetrazolium bromide (MTT) which is converted into blue or purple formazon derivative by dehydrogenases of live *M. tuberculosis* cells. The method has been evaluated for the detection of resistance of *M. tuberculosis* to first-line, second line drugs and for the detection of MDR-TB/XDR-TB strains [224, 227]. The resazurin microtitre assay is based on oxidation of resazurin by a growing culture of *M. tuberculosis* in the presence of anti-TB drugs [214, 216]. The MIC is determined as the lowest concentration of the drug that prevents change in the color of the redox indicator. The method has been used for the detection of resistance of *M. tuberculosis* strains to first-line and second-line drugs and for the detection of MDR-TB/XDR-TB strains [226-228].

The phage-based assays are another alternative for resource-poor developing countries for the detection and DST of *M. tuberculosis* from clinical specimens. These assays use different mycobacteriophages to infect live tubercle bacilli and detect the presence/growth of *M. tuberculosis* by using phage amplification assay or production of light in the absence or presence of anti-TB drug(s) [216, 229-231]. The more sensitive method based on detection of light uses luciferase reporter mycobacteriophages such as phAE142. Viable *M. tuberculosis* growing in presence of anti-TB drug and infected with phage phAE142 emit light in the presence of luciferin and are identified as drug-resistant strains [230, 231]. Some phage-based assays are also available commercially (FAST Plaque TB-Response assay). However, unlike MODS test, NR or CRI assays, phage-based assays have not yet been endorsed by WHO due to insufficient evidence of their performance in clinical settings.

6B. Molecular Diagnosis of Drug-Resistant TB, MDR-TB and XDR-TB

Conventional (phenotypic) methods for DST of *M. tuberculosis* are tedious, labor-intensive and time-consuming, typically reporting results in 1-2 weeks. The growing problem of MDR-TB prompted WHO to initiate STOP TB strategy under which universal access to diagnosis and treatment of MDR-TB was declared a priority with a focus on MDR-TB detection [232]. Molecular (genotypic) methods detect resistance associated mutations in target genes of *M. tuberculosis* and usually provide results within 1-2 days. Furthermore, these tests can be performed on clinical isolates of *M. tuberculosis* as well as on smear-positive and sometimes also on smear-negative clinical samples, allowing rapid identification of drug-resistant TB, MDR-TB and XDR-TB [37, 179, 233]. Application of a molecular diagnostic test in AFB smear-positive TB patients reduces time to detection of MDR-TB resulting in prompt placement of such patients on appropriate therapy. Rapid detection of smear-positive pulmonary TB patients infected with drug-resistant, MDR and XDR *M. tuberculosis* strains also helps in rapid isolation of such patients to arrest further transmission of infection to health care workers and other close contacts of TB patients [38, 179, 234]. Another advantage is easier handling of specimens since DNA extraction procedures render clinical material non-infectious allowing further analysis outside biosafety conditions.

Although genotypic methods have been developed for all first-line and many second-line and third-line drugs, rapid detection of RIF resistance is most feasible since 90-95% RIF-resistant strains contain mutations in 81-bp RRDR of the *rpoB* gene [78-80]. Since 85-90% RIF-resistant *M. tuberculosis* isolates are also additionally resistant to INH, detection of RIF resistance directly in clinical specimens by molecular tests (such as Xpert MTB/RIF) also identifies majority of MDR-TB strains [181, 199]. For other first-line drugs (INH, EMB and PZA), resistance conferring mechanisms are complex due to involvement of several gene loci and due to the diversity of mutations (insertions, deletions, missense or nonsense mutations) that are found in each locus among clinical *M. tuberculosis* strains [78-80]. Furthermore, the frequency of these mutations also depends on the genotype of *M. tuberculosis* strain and the ethnic origin of TB patients from whom these strains are isolated. Due to these reasons, the sensitivity of resistance detection varies considerably among *M. tuberculosis* strains isolated from different geographical locations. Despite these limitations, region-specific molecular methods have been developed for the detection of majority of drug-resistant strains. Molecular assays targeting multiple gene loci have also been developed recently to screen for mutations in several genes conferring resistance to different anti-TB drugs in a single test [78-80, 178-180]. However, most molecular methods do not detect all resistant strains and there is also a risk of incorrectly identifying some phenotypically susceptible strains as resistant strains due to silent or neutral mutations in target genes [117]. Extensive or complete genome sequencing in recent years has allowed detection of resistance conferring mutations in multiple target genes in drug-resistant *M. tuberculosis* strains leading to identification of MDR-TB and XDR-TB strains [93-95]. However, complete genome sequencing is still regarded as technically demanding and is not practical for detection of all resistance conferring mutations in target genes directly in clinical specimens.

Several methods have been developed and evaluated for the detection of mutations in target genes of *M. tuberculosis* conferring resistance to various drugs. Some of these methods such as PCR-restriction fragment length polymorphism (PCR-RFLP) and multiplex allele-specific PCR (MAS-PCR)-based assays are of limited use as they are time consuming, technically demanding and usually detect dominant mutations at single codons in target genes conferring resistance to only one anti-TB drug in each assay. The PCR-RFLP has been mostly used for detection of *katG315* and *embB306* mutations which occur in ~50-95% and 25-70% of INH resistant and EMB-resistant *M. tuberculosis* strains, respectively [37, 235-237]. Similarly, multiple MAS-PCR assays have to be performed for dominant mutation(s) in each target gene for individual drugs and still detect only a fraction of all mutations for a particular drug [238-240]. Methods that detect resistance to multiple drugs including detection of MDR-TB and/or XDR-TB strains in a single test are briefly described here.

Real-time PCR (rt-PCR) assays have been developed for rapid detection of MDR-TB strains in clinical specimens and culture isolates of *M. tuberculosis* by detecting dominant mutations in target genes conferring resistance to INH and RIF by using fluorogenic probes [241-243]. However, these assays are limited by the number of probe primers that can be effectively used in a single assay. To circumvent this problem, assays have been developed recently involving high-resolution melting curve (HRMC) analysis of rt-PCR amplicons of target regions of resistance conferring genes [244]. The method is simple, rapid, closed-tube and well suited for simultaneous detection of several mutations in resistance conferring target genes. The HRMC-based method has been successfully used for the detection of mutations in RRDR and N-terminal regions of the *rpoB* gene conferring resistance to RIF, *katG315* and regulatory region of *inhA* gene conferring resistance to INH, *rpsL* and *rrs* genes conferring resistance to SM and KAN/AMI/CAP and *gyrA* gene region conferring resistance to FQs in *M. tuberculosis* strains [245, 246]. Simultaneous detection of these mutations detects MDR-TB/XDR-TB strains. A novel quantitative rt-PCR assay developed recently detects drug-resistant, MDR- and XDR-TB strains by targeting *rrs* gene [247]. The genomic DNA of drug-susceptible strains of *M. tuberculosis* killed in the presence of anti-TB drugs is rendered unamplifiable by using propidium monoazide DNA binding dye that can penetrate damaged bacterial cells. The drug-resistant strains exhibit significant increase in threshold cycle time values during quantitative rt-PCR assays compared with drug-susceptible strains and the DST results for both, first-line and second-line drugs become available within 3 days [247].

PCR amplification of target region of resistance conferring gene(s) followed by sequencing or pyrosequencing of amplicons has also been used for the detection of drug-resistance of *M. tuberculosis* clinical isolates from solid/liquid cultures as well as directly from clinical specimens [248-251]. Direct DNA sequencing of gene target is practical if majority of drug-resistant strains contain mutations in a small region of a single target gene (RRDR of *rpoB* gene for RIF resistance) or target gene is small (*pncA* for PZA resistance) or majority of resistant strains contain mutations at one or few gene codons/regions (*katG315* and *inhA* regulatory region for INH resistance and *embB306*, *embB406* and *embB497* for EMB resistance) [78-80]. Targeted DNA sequencing and pyrosequencing have been used for the detection of mutations in target genes conferring resistance to first-line and important second-line drugs for the detection of MDR-TB and XDR-TB strains [248-251]. One study using direct DNA sequencing analysis in sputum samples reported the sensitivity of 64%, 96%, 69%, 100% and 50% for the detection of *M. tuberculosis* resistant to INH, RIF, EMB, PZA, and INH + RIF (MDR-TB), respectively, with high specificity [248]. Furthermore, many smear-negative culture positive and smear-negative culture-negative (but clinically highly suspected) specimens, yielded interpretable results. The short turnaround time combined with multilocus sequencing of several isolates in parallel makes pyrosequencing a very attractive method for drug resistance screening in *M. tuberculosis*. One study described simultaneous detection of mutations associated with resistance to INH, RIF, EMB, KAN, AMI, CAP and OFX among 290 clinical isolates of *M. tuberculosis* using seven pyrosequencing assays for *rpoB, katG, embB, rrs,* and *gyrA* gene regions and the promoter regions of *inhA* and *eis*. The pyrosequencing method demonstrated high specificity (100%) and sensitivity (94.6%) for detection of MDR-TB as well as high specificity (99.3%) and sensitivity (86.9%) for detection of XDR-TB [251].

Recent advances in sequencing technology also allow extensive targeted sequencing as well as complete genome analysis for detection of resistance conferring mutations in multiple gene targets for the detection of MDR and XDR *M. tuberculosis* strains [93-95]. Whole genome sequencing of serial *M. tuberculosis* isolates from patients during therapy have revealed transient coexistence of multiple mutants in the same sputum sample even though only a single type of mutant was ultimately selected. These findings suggest heteroresistance as a common feature of *M. tuberculosis* population and clonal selection of low-cost drug-resistant mutations [252, 253]. These studies have also identified compensatory adaptive mutations in additional genes in drug-resistant strains containing well-known resistance conferring mutations in major targets of anti-TB drugs [95, 127, 253]. Although desirable, direct application of whole genome sequencing is not yet practical with clinical specimens due to the current requirement of substantial amounts of genomic DNA for whole genome sequence analysis. However, with rapidly advancing sequencing technology, whole genome sequencing directly in clinical specimens may become feasible in the near future.

The reverse hybridization-based line probe assays (LiPAs) are PCR-based methods that simultaneously detect infection with *M. tuberculosis* and resistance to one or more anti-TB drugs [254-256]. The LiPAs were initially developed as simple and rapid molecular tests for detection of mutations conferring resistance to RIF as they are easy to perform and the results are easy to interpret [107, 257]. More recently, LiPAs have also been developed for detection of mutations conferring resistance to RIF and INH [258, 259], PZA [260, 261], FQs [260, 262, 263] as well as FQs, EMB and injectable agents (KAN/AMI/CAP) simultaneously [264] in both, culture isolates of *M. tuberculosis* as well as directly in clinical specimens. Some of these tests have been developed in-house while others are also available commercially. Three LiPAs are available commercially. The INNO-LiPA Rif TB assay detects the presence of *M. tuberculosis* and its resistance to RIF only. The GenoType MTBDR*plus* assay detects the presence of *M. tuberculosis* and its resistance to both, RIF and INH (MDR-TB). The GenoType MTBDR*sl* assay detects the presence of *M. tuberculosis* and its resistance to EMB, FQs and KAN/AMI/CAP and is used (together with GenoType MTBDR*plus* assay) to predict XDR-TB status of MDR-TB strains (Table 6.1). The INNO-LiPA Rif TB and GenoType MTBDR*plus* assays have been endorsed by WHO for rapid detection of MDR-TB strains [265].

The INNO-LiPA Rif. TB assay detects *M. tuberculosis* and its resistance to RIF due to mutations in RRDR of the *rpoB* gene [257]. Since RIF resistance is also accompanied by INH resistance in regions with a high prevalence of MDR-TB, the assay can also predict MDR status of ~85-90% *M. tuberculosis* strains in HIV-seronegative individuals [78-80]. The INNO-LiPA Rif. TB assay has been applied on culture isolates and also directly on clinical specimens. The pooled sensitivity of ~93% and ~65% have been reported for the detection of *M. tuberculosis* from smear-positive and smear-negative sputum samples, respectively with specificity values ranging from 81% to 94% [266-269]. The pooled sensitivity for the detection of RIF resistance in smear-positive sputum samples has been reported to range from 88% to 97% and from 77% to 99% for smear-negative samples [266-269].

The Genotype MTBDR*plus* assay detects RIF resistance due to mutations in RRDR of the *rpoB* gene and also simultaneously detects mutations at *katG315* and the regulatory region of *inhA* gene for INH resistance. Concomitant detection of RIF and INH resistance identifies MDR *M. tuberculosis* in cluture isolates as well as directly in sputum samples [258]. The Genotype MTBDR*plus* assay has also been evaluated extensively for the detection of *M. tuberculosis* and to diagnose RIF and INH resistance and MDR-TB [254-256]. The sensitivity of the test for detection of *M. tuberculosis* in smear-positive samples ranges from 78% to 98% depending upon the specimen's bacillary burden but is lower for smear-negative pulmonary and extrapulmonary specimens [254, 258, 270-272]. The sensitivity of the test for extrapulmonary specimens, particularly smear-negative samples has been improved recently by a modified version of the test [273, 274]. The pooled sensitivity of Genotype MTBDR*plus* assay for RIF resistance is reported as ~98% in culture confirmed cases as well as in smear-positive sputum samples. The pooled sensitivity of the test for INH resistance is ~89% in culture confirmed cases but lower in clinical specimens. The sensitivity of the assay for simultaneous detection of RIF + INH resistance (MDR-TB) in culture isolates and smear-positive sputum samples has also been reported as ~85-90% in various studies [254-256, 258, 270-274]. The Genotype MTBDR*plus* assay has been simplified recently by omitting probe for specific detection of uncommon (AGC to ACA) mutation at *katG315* and two probes for detection of specific mutations at -8 position of regulatory region of *inhA* gene. However, the performance of the test is not affected as these mutations are still detected by lack of hybridization of respective wild-type probes [273, 274].

The Genotype MTBDR*sl* assay detects resistance to FQs, injectable second-line drugs KAN, AMI and CAP and to EMB by interrogating mutations at *gyrA* codons 90-94 most commonly observed in FQ-resistant strains, mutations at *rrs* nucleotides 1401 and 1484 commonly observed in KAN/AMI/CAP-resistant strains and mutations at *embB306* commonly observed in EMB-resistant *M. tuberculosis* strains [78-80]. The combination of Genotype MTBDR*sl* and Genotype MTBDR*plus* thus allows detection of *M. tuberculosis* infection and XDR-TB in culture isolates and also directly in clinical specimens [258, 264]. The pooled sensitivity of Genotype MTBDR*sl* for detection of resistance to FQs, KAN, AMI and CAP was reported as 85%, 83%, 90% and 87%, respectively [275-277]. Similarly high sensitivity was also noted when the test was applied directly on smear-positive sputum samples [277-280]. The high sensitivity combined with high specificity of the Genotype MTBDR*sl* assay makes it suitable for rapid screening of culture isolates for XDR-TB. The application of Genotype MTBDR*sl* has been shown to shorten the time to diagnosis of XDR-TB in high prevalence settings [280]. Another commercial line probe assay that has become available recently has four strips designed to detect *M. tuberculosis* infection and resistance to INH plus RIF (MDR-TB) (strip 1), more extensive coverage for greater sensitivity for detection of resistance to INH (strip 2), resistance to PZA (strip 3) and resistance to FQs (strip 4) [259]. The sensitivity for detection of resistance to RIF, INH, PZA and FQs for culture isolates was reported as 99%, 91%, 90%, and 93%, respectively [259]. The performance of this assay has not yet been evaluated directly on sputum or other clinical specimens.

Although PZA has important sterilizing effect and reduces relapse rates in
ents treated with RIF-containing regimens, the DST for PZA is not
rmined routinely due to optimal activity of the drug at lower pH or may
uce unreliable results [287, 288]. Hence, most drug resistance surveys do
include data on PZA resistance [24]. Monoresistant strains of *M.*
rculosis to PZA have been described and are associated with poorer
cal outcome despite treatment for longer period (9 months) with at least 6
ths of treatment with RIF-containing regimens [289].

Monoresistance to RIF, though rare in general, occurs more frequently
g patients with HIV-coinfection or other underlying conditions [102-
However, the possibility of under-detection of INH resistance should be
tained if DST is carried out without adequate quality assurance or by
cular methods that have lower sensitivity for detecting INH resistance
. Treatment of infections caused by RIF-resistant *M. tuberculosis* strains
sociated with poorer outcome and higher relapse rates even when
nent with 4 drugs is continued for 9 months [44, 145, 282, 287]. This is
urprising since RIF is the most effective drug against non-replicating
ant form of *M. tuberculosis* (persisters) which are mainly responsible for
nent failure and disease relapse. Extending the duration of therapy to 12
s has been shown to improve outcome [291].

reatment of infections with polydrug-resistant (INH + EMB or INH +
or EMB + PZA or INH + EMB + PZA) *M. tuberculosis* strains requires
l clinical evaluation but can also be successfully managed with extended
nent (~18 months) with remaining first-line drug(s) in combination
y with other bactericidal agents (FQs and injectable agents) with/without
second-line agents [282, 287, 291]. However, disease relapse occurs
frequently and treatment failure in new cases with preexisting polydrug
nce has been reported to be nearly 21% compared to 8% for monodrug-
nt TB, particularly when RIF was used for <5 months [287]. If DST
are not reliable or if sputum sample was collected several weeks before
esults became available, the possibility of development of additional
nce should be considered, particularly for FQs as resistance to this class
gs may develop after a short period of exposure. If patients remain
smear-positive without clinical improvement, at least three new drugs
be added or a full MDR-TB regimen should be considered to prevent
development of resistance.

though initial outbreaks of MDR-TB were mainly reported among HIV-
ted patients and were associated with very high mortality and disease
rates, advances in rapid diagnosis, aggressive therapy with several

Chapter VII

Treatment of Drug-Resistant TB, MDR-TB and XDR-TB

Fully susceptible TB is defined as active disease caused by a clinical *M. tuberculosis* isolate that fails to grow *in vitro* in the presence of any first-line anti-TB drug. As stated above, treatment of susceptible TB is highly effective (≥95% cure rate) by combination therapy with all four first-line drugs in the initiation phase of two months and with INH and RIF in the continuation phase of four months [43-45]. Active disease caused by a strain of *M. tuberculosis* that grows in the presence of one anti-TB drug *in vitro* is classified as monodrug-resistant TB while resistance to various combinations of first-line drugs excluding INH and RIF is called polydrug-resistant TB. However, resistance to INH and RIF with or without additional drug resistance is clinically more significant as these two drugs represent the most powerful anti-TB agents currently available and is defined as MDR-TB [5, 6]. Extensively drug-resistant TB, recognized more recently, is defined as infection with an MDR-TB strain that is additionally resistant to a FQ and one of three (KAN, AMI or CAP) injectable agent [6, 21]. Several factors, such as initial drug resistance, organ affected, presence of lung cavity, time to detection on automated liquid mycobacterial cultures, infection with more virulent (W-Beijing genotype) strains of *M. tuberculosis*, HIV status of TB patient and availability of several drugs to which the *M. tuberculosis* isolate is susceptible, determine the treatment outcome [44, 56, 145, 281].

7A. Treatment of Drug-Resistant TB, MDR-TB and XDR-TB in HIV-Seronegative Adults

Resistance profile of the infecting *M. tuberculosis* strain is the single most important factor as treatment regimens and duration of treatment are devised accordingly [44, 145]. Consequently, monodrug-resistant/polydrug-resistant TB is generally easier to treat and cure more effectively than MDR-TB while XDR-TB is considered as the most difficult form of TB to treat. The number and combination of available first-line and second-line/third-line drugs (listed in Table 3.1) used and treatment strategy for infections caused by *M. tuberculosis* strains with different resistance patterns are shown in Table 7.1.

Resistance of clinical *M. tuberculosis* isolates to SM is described frequently, however, SM is no longer used as a first-line drug and is usually replaced by EMB in combination therapy [44]. Mono-resistance to EMB is infrequent and treatment duration and risk of treatment failure for EMB-resistant TB is same as for fully susceptible TB since EMB is used only during initiation phase and can be easily replaced by highly active injectable Group II agents or oral FQs [44, 45, 282]. Monodrug-resistance to INH occurs more frequently [24, 44].

The outcome of INH-resistant TB with daily 9-month regimen of RIF, PZA and EMB in settings with low TB rates is favorable while treatment outcomes are relatively poor in settings with high incidence of TB and drug-resistant TB [67, 283-285].

A meta-analysis has shown that daily oral therapy with regimens containing RIF together with several other effective drugs, and an injectable agent (KAN, AMI or CAP), for a total duration of >6 months is associated with lower rates of treatment failure, disease relapse or acquired resistance to additional anti-TB drugs [286].

However, under-detection of RIF resistance must be carefully excluded, which may be easily missed for low-level but clinically significant RIF-resistant *M. tuberculosis* strains by broth-based automated systems [117].

Table 7.1. Treatment regimens and minimum duration of treatment for patients with different patterns of drug-resistant TB, MDR-TB and XDR-TB

Resistance of M. tuberculosis strain to anti-TB drug(s)[a]	Disease status	Drugs to be included in appropriate therapy regimens	Minimum treatment duration (months)	Desirable number of drugs for effective treatment
None	Susceptible TB	INH, RIF, PZA, EMB	6	4
EMB or SM	Monodrug-resistant TB	INH, RIF, PZA, Group 2 or 3	6	4
PZA	Monodrug-resistant TB	INH, RIF, EMB, Group 2 or 3	6 to 9	4
INH	Monodrug-resistant TB	RIF, PZA, EMB, Group 2 or 3	6 to 9	4
RIF	Monodrug-resistant TB	INH, PZA, EMB, Group 2 + 3	9 to 12	4 to 5
INH, SM or EMB	Polydrug-resistant TB	RIF, PZA, EMB, Group 2 ± 3	6 to 9	4 to 5
INH, PZA	Polydrug-resistant TB	RIF, EMB, Group 2 + 3	6 to 9	4 to 5
INH, EMB, PZA	Polydrug-resistant TB	RIF, Group 2 + 3 ± 4	6 to 9	4 to 5
INH, RIF	MDR-TB	PZA, EMB, Group 2 + 3 ± 4	18 to 24	5 to 6
INH, RIF, EMB	MDR-TB	PZA, Group 2 + 3 ± 4 ± surgery	18 to 24	5 to 6
INH, RIF, PZA	MDR-TB	EMB, Group 2 + 3 + 4 ± surgery	24	5 to 7
INH, RIF, PZA, EMB	MDR-TB	Group 2 + 3 + 4 ± surgery	24	5 to 7
INH, RIF, PZA, EMB, Group 2	MDR-TB	Group 2 + 3 + 4 ± surgery	>24	5 to 7
INH, RIF, PZA, EMB, Group 3	MDR-TB	Group 2 + 3 + 4 ± surgery	>24	5 to 7
INH, RIF, Group 2 + Goup 3	XDR-TB	Group 2[b] + 3[c] + 4 + 5 + surgery	>24	5 to 7

[illegible] INH, isoniazid; RIF, rifampicin; Group 2, includes injectable agents such as kanamycin, [illegible] moxifloxacin; Group 4, active drugs and close monitoring of patients in mid 1990s considerably improved clinical outcome [44, 292]. Treatment of MDR-TB is still lengthy, much more expensive, toxic and is associated with higher rates of clinical failure and disease relapse [36-38, 293-295]. Successful management of MDR-TB requires DST for first- and second-line drugs, and monitoring of patients for bacteriological (sputum smear and culture) and radiological improvement and adverse drug reactions. In developing countries, treatment of MDR-TB is difficult due to delayed diagnosis, lack of universal availability of DST facilities and non-availability of adequate supplies of second-line drugs. Both CDC and WHO recommend DST for first-line and important second-line drugs (by molecular methods, if available) and treatment regimens should include all available first-line and several most active second-line drugs (Table 7.1). Recent advances in the development of cost-effective methods for detection and DST of *M. tuberculosis* strains have resulted in wider availability of these methods in resource-poor settings [213-216].

Two basic treatment approaches are mainly used. Either standardized treatment regimens are designed based on representative drug-resistance surveillance data or individualized regimens are tailored on the basis of patient's previous history of anti-TB treatment and DST results [36-38, 291, 293-295]. Although demanding, individualized treatment has better outcome while inadequately designed standardized regimens that do not match representative drug resistance patterns do not perform satisfactorily [291, 296]. Previous use of a second-line drug for more than a month was found to be associated with reduced efficacy even when DST results indicated *in vitro* susceptibility [297]. Treatment recommendations for MDR-TB include an intensive phase of at least 6-8 months (4 months after culture conversion) with 5-6 effective drugs that include PZA, a FQ (preferably a new generation FQ like LFX, GFX or MFX), an injectable agent (KAN, AMI or CAP/VIO) and 2-3 other second line drugs, preferably including ETA or PTA and CS or TZD (Table 7.1). With good clinical response, the injectable agent may be discontinued after 8 months of therapy, however, the continuation phase with 4 effective drugs should continue for a minimum of 20 months (18 months after culture conversion) [291, 294, 298]. PAS or group 5 agents may also be included if resistance or toxicity concerns preclude inclusion of sufficient number of effective drugs. CFZ has been successfully used in Bangladesh and LZD at doses that are effective but reduce adverse drug reactions has also been used [298-300]. EMB and high dose INH may also be included in MDR-TB regimens as additional drugs in some cases [291, 301].

Adverse reactions occur frequently and pose a challenge in the treatment of MDR-TB [36, 293, 302, 303]. To minimize adverse effects, only one second-line oral agent such as ETA/PTA may be added in ascending or multiple smaller daily doses to therapy regimens containing PZA (and EMB if still effective), FQ (preferably LFX/MFX) and an injectable (KAN, AMI or CAP/VIO) agent. Once the patients can tolerate smaller doses, a single daily dose may be given and is to be followed by addition of another second-line agent. Regular (at least once a month) sputum-smear examination, culture and DST predict response to treatment and should be carried out until sputum culture conversion (culture negative status) has been achieved [304-306]. This is neccessitated by bacteriostatic nature and lower efficacy of many second-line drugs that are used for the treatment of MDR-TB. Surgery could also be considered in specific cases when insufficient number of second-line drugs are available and the patient has localized lesions and can tolerate surgery [307-309].

The total duration of treatment for MDR-TB is usually guided by the timing of sputum culture conversion after initiation of therapy and therapy should continue for at least 18 months after culture conversion [304]. The outcome of MDR-TB treatment is highly variable. The proportion of patients with favorable outcome has been reported to vary from <40% to ~97% in different studies [36, 293, 310]. These variations are partly due to outcome definitions for treatment success and failure. A recent meta-analysis of patients with multidrug-resistant pulmonary TB found pooled treatment success of 75% compared to failure/relapse/death (but excluding default) and patients who died during treatment were more likely to be older, HIV-coinfected, had more extensive disease, previous exposure to a higher number of anti-TB drugs and/or had prior history of treatment with second-line drugs [310]. Recurrence of MDR-TB has also been reported among patients who completed treatment but apparently were not completely cured. The use of PZA, a new generation FQ (LFX/GFX/MFX), ETA/PTA, KAN and CS as part of multidrug regimen was associated with treatment success. Furthermore, treatment outcome was superior when Group 5 drugs were not used or only 1 Group 5 drug was used. The treatment success rate was also higher in patients who received 7-8 months of initial intensive phase with 5 drugs and a continuation phase with 4 drugs resulting in total treatment duration of up to 24 months [310]. However, one study has shown that shorter duration of treatment of MDR-TB patients not treated previously with second-line drugs is feasible. Treatment of HIV-seronegative Bangladeshi MDR-TB patients in a 9-month regimen containing PZA, EMB, GFX (OFX was less effective), CFZ with a 4-month intensive initiation phase additionally containing KAN, PTA and high-dose INH resulted in a relapse free cure rate of ~90% with manageable adverse drug reactions [299]. This study showed that some MDR-TB patients may be successfully treated with a shorter regimen than currently recommended by WHO [311]. Successful treatment of MDR-TB also avoids the generation of XDR-TB.

Although principles of treatment and management of XDR-TB are the same as for MDR-TB, successful treatment of XDR-TB is much more difficult even in developed countries while in resource-poor developing countries, XDR-TB is virtually an untreatable disease [38-40, 312-314]. The management of XDR-TB is much more complex and no single strategy is likely to fit all situations. This is because the remaining second-line and other drugs are ineffective in efficiently killing tubercle bacilli of different metabolic state (actively dividing, semi-dormant or dormant) and in different environments (extracellular or in phagosomes inside macrophages) in TB patients. Since the definition of XDR-TB is not based on resistance to all FQs and all injectable agents, treatment of XDR-TB should include an appropriate injectable agent (cross-rersistance between KAN, AMI, CAP and VIO is not complete) and a FQ (some OFX-resistant strains remain susceptible to MFX) based on DST profile or prior treatment history. Also, all Group 4 agents that have not been used extensively in previous regimens or those that are likely to be effective and two to several Group 5 agents should be included in therapy regimens [38-40, 312-314]. Other experimental drugs have also been used occasionally for the treatment of XDR-TB patients with varying degree of success [74, 315, 316].

Similar to MDR-TB treatment, close bacteriological and radiological monitoring of patients for clinical improvement, complete adherence to treatment and proper management of adverse drug reactions improve prognosis [38-40, 312, 313]. For pulmonary TB patients with localized disease and limited lung tissue damage, surgical resection may lower bacterial burden and improve clinical outcome [307-309]. As with MDR-TB, addition of PZA, EMB or SM in multidrug regimens improves prognosis in patients with XDR-TB [40, 317]. Patients who fail to undergo sputum culture conversion within 6 months of starting treatment with several anti-TB drugs are more likely to fail therapy than those patients who achieve sputum culture conversion during this initial intensive phase of treatment. However, the prognosis of XDR-TB is generally poorer than for MDR-TB and patients are more likely to fail treatment [38-40, 67, 312].

7B. Treatment of Drug-Resistant TB in Children

The above guidelines are intended for the treatment of adult TB patients with drug-resistant TB/MDR-TB/XDR-TB. Drug-resistant TB in children is usually transmitted from close contacts with adult pulmonary source cases and information for treatment of pediatric population is very limited. Childhood MDR-TB/XDR-TB is an emerging global epidemic but children with TB often have a negative culture due to paucibacillary load in sputum/other respiratory or gastric specimens making management more difficult [21, 318, 319]. Often, drug-resistant TB is suspected if there is known contact with an adult source case of MDR-TB/XDR-TB. However, with recent advances in molecular diagnostic methods, more children are likely to be identified and will require treatment with second-line and other anti-TB drugs [318-320]. Children usually differ from adults in the manner in which drugs are administered, metabolized, drug-drug interactions occur and in the ways adverse drug reactions are experienced. However, information on pharmacokinetic and pharmacodynamic properties of second-line and other available anti-TB drugs, adverse effects and drug interactions in pediatric populations is very limited [320]. Furthermore, growth and development needs of children should be monitored during therapy and dose adjustments may be needed for weight gain during the long treatment period. Treatment of HIV-coinfected children with MDR-TB/XDR-TB is even more complex due to additional problems of poor drug absorption and drug-drug interactions with concomitant antiretroviral therapy [321]. Also MDR tuberculous meningitis in children has very high mortality [322].

7C. Treatment of Drug-Resistant TB in HIV-Coinfected Patients

The HIV coinfection in patients with drug-resistant TB, MDR-TB or XDR-TB poses particular diagnostic and therapeutic challenges. The WHO guidelines recommend starting antiretroviral therapy in HIV-coinfected individuals soon (within 2-8 weeks for patients with CD4 counts of <350) after the diagnosis of MDR-TB [291]. As smear microscopy for AFB is the main and sometimes the only rapid method used for TB diagnosis in poor, developing countries where HIV-TB coinfection is common, the diagnosis of pulmonary TB is often delayed due to paucibacillary load in sputum samples and atypical presentation [4, 10, 50]. Even when the disease is diagnosed early, the treatment is complicated by the requirement of taking large number of drugs each day for a very long time (~2 years), poor absorption of anti-TB drugs due to vomiting and/or diarrhea and emergence of immune reconstitution inflammatory syndrome characterized by worsening of clinical symptoms and appearance of new TB lesions [4, 10, 50, 323]. Potentially severe drug-drug interactions between RIF and protease/nonnucleoside reverse transcriptase inhibitors pose serious challenges to effective treatment of drug-resistant TB [51, 52]. Although substitution of RBU for RIF has fewer problematic drug-drug interactions, however, the regimen becomes prohibitively expensive for resource-poor settings [53, 57].

The treatment of MDR-TB in HIV-coinfected patients is further complicated by excessive toxicity of some drugs (e.g., thiacetazone) and additive adverse drug effects between anti-retroviral agents and second-line anti-TB drugs among patients undergoing concomitant anti-retroviral and anti-TB therapy [4, 10, 50]. Despite these limitations, recent developments in rapid diagnosis of MDR-TB, aggressive therapy with several active drugs, close radiological and bacteriological (for sputum smear and culture) monitoring of patients have reduced mortality rates in HIV-coinfected TB patients. Rapid initiation of MDR-TB treatment with appropriate empiric regimens at centers equipped with specialized expertise to manage several complex modalities is essential for achieving good treatment outcome [324]. A comprehensive community-based treatment and care program with a referral center of expertise in Lesotho, South Africa managed to reduce early mortality from MDR-TB in HIV-coinfected persons from >70% to 30% [325-327]. However, the outcome of XDR-TB in HIV-coinfected individuals generally remains dismal with mortality rates of ~80% within few weeks of diagnosis [41, 328].

Chapter VIII

New Drugs for the Treatment of TB and Drug-Resistant TB

The increasing prevalence of MDR-TB and XDR-TB is threatening to mirror the situation of pre-antibiotic era when the clinicians mainly relied upon fresh air, host immunity, rest and good nutrition for the treatment of active disease patients [27]. There is a desperate need for new compounds to treat drug-resistant TB by regimens that will be tolerated better and will shorten treatment duration. In the short-term, currently available drugs already approved for human use will be used in novel treatment strategies to maximize outcome of drug-resistant TB [70, 295, 329]. In the long term, more potent drugs with novel mechanism of action will be required for rapid and more effective treatment of MDR-TB/XDR-TB [330]. A number of novel drugs are currently in various stages of clinical development and will hopefully become available in the near future [331-334]. Effective new drugs should have potency greater that INH against actively dividing bacteria and potency greater than RIF for non-replicating persistent tubercle bacilli in order to shorten the treatment duration of drug sensitive active TB to ~3 months. A brief description of new uses for existing drugs and some novel drugs under development is given below.

8A. Clinical Re-evaluation of Existing Drugs

Several existing drugs are being re-evaluated to simplify and shorten the duration of drug-susceptible TB and to increase the efficacy of treatment for drug-resistant TB and MDR-TB. These include the use of high-dose INH and RIF, substitution of RIF by RPE or RBU, increasing the potency of PZA and repositioning of third-generation FQs, linezolid, phenothiazines and carbapenems in treatment regimens.

Nearly 15-20% of INH-resistant *M. tuberculosis* strains contain mutations only in *inhA* regulatory region and exhibit low-level of resistance to INH but high-level cross-resistance to thioamides (ETA/PTA) [80, 169, 317]. Since the currently recommended dose of INH (5 mg/kg) can be effectively increased 2-3 times (10-15 mg/kg), high-dose INH therapy has been shown to effectively overcome the problem of cross-resistance to thioamides in the treatment of MDR-TB patients. In one study, high-dose INH regimen reduced bacterial burden, making sputum of MDR-TB patients smear-negative more rapidly and more often, together with radiological improvement without increased risk of INH-related toxicity [301]. Due to its low cost, reliable DST and favorable pharmacokinetic profile, high-dose INH has been used in several countries with encouraging results [335, 336]. However, high-dose INH therapy is currently not included in the WHO guidelines for the treatment of MDR-TB patients [291].

RIF and PZA are the main sterilizing drugs in the current standard treatment regimen and improving their activity may help in shortening the treatment duration for drug-susceptible TB [43-45, 337]. The currently used daily adult dose of RIF (600 mg), likely chosen due to high cost of the drug during its inception, is rather low in some patients [338]. High-dose RIF (1200 mg) given daily doubles its EBA and is also well-tolerated by most TB patients [339, 340]. Phase II clinical trials are underway to evaluate efficacy and drug tolerance of high-dose RIF in TB patients for the possibility of shortening treatment duration to 4 months. RPE has four-times lower MIC and better pharmacokinetic properties than RIF and 5 days/week administration of RPE (10 mg/kg) along with INH and PZA for 3 months cured mice and prevented relapse while standard RIF containing regimen required 6 months [100]. However, when the same regimen supplemented with EMB was tried in humans, it was only as effective as the standard regimen [341]. RPE is also well-tolerated at higher doses (>15 mg/kg) [342]. Further studies are underway with daily, high-dose therapy with RPE for shortening treatment duration of drug-susceptible TB to ~4 months. However, high-dose RIF- or RPE-based regimens will be problematic in HIV-coinfected individuals on antiretroviral therapy due to drug-drug interactions of RIF or RPE with anti-retroviral drugs.

Another rifamycin, RBU, is also useful for the treatment of 15%-20% RIF-resistant (including some MDR-TB) strains with mutations in the *rpoB* gene as they remain susceptible to RBU [121-124]. RBU is also useful for HIV-coinfected individuals due to less problematic drug-drug interactions with protease inhibitors during anti-retroviral therapy [53]. New rifabutin analogs have also been synthesized recently that exhibit lower *in vitro* MIC values than RIF and RBU against both, RIF-susceptible and MDR-TB strains [125]. The high cost of RBU and the problem of accurate DST procedure have, however, restricted its use, particularly in developing countries.

Higher doses of PZA (>25 mg/kg) increase hepatotoxicity considerably without substantial improvements in its activity and consequently are not useful. However, concomitant administration of pyrazinoic acid through inhalation as a supplement to oral dose has been suggested as an alternative. This approach will likely lead to acidification of lung lesions which should lead to greater efficacy of the oral dose and may also be effective against most PZA-resistant strains since mutations in *pncA* causing inactivation of pyrazinamidase that converts the pro-drug PZA into pyrazinoic acid is the major mechanism conferring resistance to PZA [128-133, 337].

The FQs are generally well tolerated and offer the convenience of once daily oral dosing in combination therapy. Two 8-methoxy fluoroquinolones, MFX and GFX, are potent antibacterial agents with MIC of 0.125-0.5 mg/L and EBA approaching that of INH in patients with pulmonary TB [61, 343]. Three phase II clinical trials evaluated the efficacy of substitution of MFX for EMB in the intensive phase of treatment of sputum smear-positive pulmonary TB patients for shortening the treatment duration and have yielded variable results. The first study, carried out by the TB Trials Consortium, reported higher rates of sputum culture conversion at 4 and 6 weeks of therapy but not at week 8 in MFX-containing regimen [63]. Another study conducted in Rio de Janeiro, Brazil, reported higher rates of sputum culture conversion beginning at 2 weeks which persisted till 8 weeks in MFX-containing regimen [66]. The third study carried out in Durban, South Africa (OFLUTUB Consortium study) reported rapid elimination of viable bacteria from sputum of pulmonary TB patients in the intensive phase of standard WHO recommended 6-month regimen. [64]. The effect of replacement of INH with MFX was also evaluated in a phase II double blind, randomized controlled trial in the intensive phase of treatment of sputum smear-positive pulmonary TB patients. The conversion from positive sputum cultures at initiation of therapy to negative cultures from sputum specimens after 8 weeks of therapy occurred in 99 (60.4%) of 164 participants in MFX group versus 90 (54.9%) of 164 participants in the INH group [65]. The data showed a slight but statistically insignificant (p=0.37) increase in sputum conversion rate in MFX-containing regimen and similar number of adverse drug events in both, the FQ arm and the control arm during these studies [65].

The MFX is now in two separate phase III clinical trials for the treatment of adult patients newly diagnosed with drug-susceptible, pulmonary TB for investigation of whether treatment duration can be effectively shortened to 4 months by substitution of MFX for either EMB or INH [344, 345]. The results of these trials will determine whether MFX becomes a first-line drug for the treatment of drug-susceptible TB. A recent study involving coadministration of MFX and RIF in a murine aerosol infection model showed mild antagosim between MFX and RIF activities [346]. However, this does not compromise the effectiveness of MFX in combined drug regimens for treatment of MDR-TB.

A major concern is the frequent use of FQs as first-line therapy to treat lower respiratory tract infections (such as community-acquired pneumonia) other than tuberculosis as this can result in selection of FQ-resistant TB when TB is misdiagnosed. There are no clear international recommendations to protect FQs as effective anti-TB drugs and many countries have no national policy for ensuring the efficacy of these drugs. In some settings, published expert recommendations and clinical guidelines or unrestricted availability of antibiotics have promoted widespread use of FQs for common infections such as pneumonia and sinusitis.

The empirical FQ prescriptions are likely to be more problematic in countries with a high TB incidence since patients diagnosed with lower respiratory tract infections in such settings may, in fact, have active TB disease more often than in developed countries and the diagnosis of their active disease may be further delayed by monotherapy with FQs. Prolonged exposure of such patients to FQs may contribute to the emergence of FQ resistance in *M. tuberculosis*. Recent WHO reports suggest that ~25% of MDR-TB strains from China and India are likely to be resistant to FQs. Also, the resistance of *M. tuberculosis* strains to FQs is common in several other countries and is rapidly increasing [6, 21, 24].

One recent study showed that the risk of FQ-resistant TB was higher in patients who had received FQs for more than 10 days for lower respiratory tract infections and this trend was stronger in patients who were diagnosed with active TB disease and who were prescribed a FQ for a respiratory infection [347]. Two systematic reviews have also shown that empiric treatment of bacterial pneumonia with FQs was associated with longer delays in TB diagnosis and treatment of pulmonary TB and a higher risk of developing FQ-resistant TB in such patients [348, 349]. It has been suggested that national community acquired pneumonia guidelines should ensure rational use of FQs so that we do not lose this important class of anti-TB drugs [350].

Bactericidal activity of carbapenems (IMP and MEP) combined with CLV (inhibitor of *blaC* encoded β-lactamase) was recently shown for replicating, non-replicating and drug-resistant *M. tuberculosis* strains [73, 351, 352]. One recent study has also shown synergy between AMX-CLV in combination with MEP [74]. However, the current use of carbapenems is limited to more severe cases of MDR-TB/XDR-TB due to the requirement of parenteral administration of these drugs.

Clofazimine (CFZ), a fat-soluble riminophenazine and an established anti-leprosy agent, was initially developed as an anti-TB drug in the 1950s but its use declined soon afterward due to adverse side-effects (skin discoloration, crystal deposits of the drug in tissues and gastric intolerance) and availability of more active and safer drugs (INH, SM and PAS) [353]. The drug has recently been approved by WHO as a Group 5 drug due to its low cost and the limited choices available for the treatment of severe cases of MDR-TB [70]. A recent study carried out in Bangladesh for the treatment of MDR-TB patients showing effective application (~90% cure rate) of a 9-month regimen containing CFZ and 6 other drugs in the intensive phase of treatment has renewed interest in this drug [299].

Addition of CFZ to a multi-drug regimen containing other experimental drugs only was also found to be superior compared to a first-line regimen containing RIF, INH and PZA in a murine model of infection [354]. Recently, more potent analogs of CFZ have been synthesized that show fewer potential side effects (tissue accumulation and skin discoloration) [355, 356].

Linezolid, an oxazolidinone class of antibiotic is active against *M. tuberculosis* and has been used in multidrug regimens for the treatment of complicated cases of MDR-TB/XDR-TB [71, 72, 300, 357, 358]. However, widespread use is limited due to its high cost and toxicity over extended period as nearly 50% patients experience reduction in white cell and platelet count (meylosuppression) or peripheral/optic neuropathy [300, 359, 360]. Although cost and toxicity concerns have been somewhat reduced by using 50% of the original drug dose (600 mg/day or 300 mg twice/day), its use is still restricted to more severe cases of MDR-TB/XDR-TB due to the requirement of close monitoring for adverse events and frequent drug discontinuation [72, 300, 359-361]. One study has reported encouraging results even at the drug dose of 300 mg/day with fewer side effects [362]. Encouraged by these findings, drug companies initiated efforts that led to the development of more active and less toxic oxazolidinones which are being evaluated in clinical trials for their efficacy (see below).

An interesting approach has been used recently to increase the efficacy of thioamides (ETA and PTA) by including positive regulators of pro-drug activation in treatment regimens. ETA/PTA are prodrugs that are activated by a monoxygenase encoded by *ethA* whose espression is regulated by a repressor protein encoded by *ethR* [363, 364]. EthR inhibitors boost antibacterial activity of ETA by increasing the synthesis of EthA [316]. The efficacy of ETA and PTA has recently been boosted by including the inhibitors of EthR in treatment regimens. BDM31343 was initially identified as one such agent that decreased the effective dose of ETA by three-fold without affecting efficacy [365].

Other thiophen-2-yl-1,2,4-oxadiazoles derivatives of BDM31343 with better solubility and metabolic stability have also been synthesized as more potent EthR inhibitors that may improve the tolerability of ETA/PTA by reducing the effective dose or improve the potency of currently used drug doses [366-368].

Another approach is to use phenothiazines such as thioridazine (TDZ), an anti-epileptic drug that interferes with several metabolic pathways in *M. tuberculosis* including aerobic respiration due to inhibition of respiratory chain enzyme NADH dehydrogenase.

TDZ accumulates in macrophages and thus, enhances their killing potential for intracellular *M. tuberculosis* [369-371]. TDZ and other phenothiazines also inhibit the genetic expression as well as activity of efflux pumps that contribute to the multidrug-resistant phenotype of *M. tuberculosis* and thus, increase the efficacy of less-effective anti-TB drugs. Combination of TDZ with antibiotics thus, enhances the activity of unresponsive anti-TB drugs and contributes in the management of XDR-TB [315, 369, 371].

Table 8.1. Potential antitubercular drugs in different stages of development for the treatment of drug-susceptible TB, drug-resistant TB, MDR-TB and XDR-TB

Potential new antitubercular drug	Chemical description	Biological process inhibited	[a]MIC range (mg/L)	Current stage of development
Bedaquiline, TMC207	Diarylquinolone	ATP synthesis	0.03-0.12	Phase III
PA-824	Nitroimidazo-oxazine	Mycolic acid synthesis	0.06-0.53	Phase II
Delamanid, OPC67683	Nitroimidazo-oxazole	Mycolic acid synthesis	0.006-0.024	Phase III
SQ109	Ethylenediamine derivative	Cell wall synthesis	0.7-1.6	Phase II
PNU-100480	Oxazolidinone derivative	Protein synthesis	0.03-0.50	Phase II
AZD5847	Oxazolidinone derivative	Protein synthesis	$\leq$1.0	Phase II
FAS 20013	Sulphonylcarboxamide	Lipid/cell wall synthesis	~0.8	Phase I
BTZ043	Nitro-benzothiazinone derivative	Lipid/cell wall synthesis	0.001-0.004	Preclinical
DNB1	Dinitrobenzamide derivative	Lipid/cell wall synthesis	$\leq$0.001	Preclinical
SQ609	Dipiperidine derivative	Cell wall synthesis	$\leq$4.0	Preclinical
SQ641	Capuramycin derivative	Cell wall synthesis	~1.0	Preclinical
CPZEN-45	Caprazamycin derivative	Cell wall synthesis	1.6-6.2	Preclinical
DC-159a	New 8-methoxy-fluoroquinolone	DNA replication	0.03-1.0	Preclinical

[a]MIC, minimum inhibitory concentration

8B. New Anti-TB Drugs Under Development

Despite the problems associated with accurate DST of *M. tuberculosis* strains to some second-line and most third-line drugs, recent reports of *M. tuberculosis* strains resistant to nearly all tested antituberculars have made it very clear that there is an urgent need for a new generation of anti-TB drugs that should have good oral bioavailability and must be active against drug-resistant forms of tubercle bacilli [29-32]. Since TB is also the leading cause of death among HIV-coinfected individuals, the newer agents should also be active in combined treatment of HIV/TB coinfections with favorable pharmacokinetic drug interactions and manageable toxicities [21, 372]. Several new anti-TB drugs are at various stages of clinical evaluation and preclinical development and are listed in Table 8.1. A brief description of current status of their development is described below.

8B.1. New Drugs under Clinical Evaluation

Bedaquiline (also known as TMC207 or R207910), a diarylquinoline, being developed by Tibotec in collaboration with TB alliance, has a novel mechanism of action which makes it highly potent against both, drug-susceptible and drug-resistant strains of *M. tuberculosis*. The drug binds to subunit c of ATP synthase (encoded by *atpE*) and inhibits the proton transfer chain of ATP synthase leading to inadequate synthesis of ATP [373-375]. The MIC ranges between 0.03-0.12 mg/L against both, drug-susceptible and drug-resistant strains of *M. tuberculosis* residing extracellularly and inside macrophages (Table 8.1) but the drug is not active on human mitochondrial ATP synthase [373, 375, 376]. Importantly, bedaquiline, though derived from quinolones, has no inhibitoy effect on DNA gyrase of *M. tuberculosis*. The bactericidal activity of bedaquiline against nonreplicating bacteria points to its possible role in shortening treatment regimens. The EBA of bedaquiline at a dose of 400 mg in pulmonary TB (including HIV-coinfected) patients is comparable to that of INH and RIF but with a delayed onset. The killing of actively dividing tubercle bacilli is initially slow and time-dependent as it starts a few days after treatment has commenced due to gradual reduction of ATP concentration but becomes more rapid as treatment continues while killing is more rapid and concentration dependent for non-replicating intracellular bacilli (persisters) due to their already lower ATP levels [376, 377].

Bedaquiline is administered orally, its serum concentration is higher when the drug is taken along with food and is metabolized by the hepatic CYP450 enyzymes suggesting the possibility of unfavorable interactions with RIF and its usefulness for the treatment of RIF-resistant TB and MDR-TB [378, 379]. However, it shows synergistic activity with PZA and combination therapy with regimens containing PZA is highly effective. Single-dose bedaquiline is well tolerated and its serum concentration is not affected by concomitant administration of CYP450 inducing antiretroviral drug efavirenz [380]. Pharmakokinetic studies in mice have shown that bedaquiline (TMC207) has long plasma and tissue half-life and good tissue penetration. Furthermore, substitution of INH or RIF with TMC207 in regimens also containing PZA cleared the infection in lungs of all mice (complete culture conversion) after 2 months of treatment [381]. Similarly, combination therapy of guinea pigs with TMC207, RIF and PZA for only 8 weeks also reduced bacterial load in the lungs to undetectable levels and relapse rates in treated animals were slightly lower (but statistically insignificant) than in another group of animals which had been treated with RIF, INH and PZA for 24 weeks [382]. A combination of second-line regimens containing TMC207, PZA and MFX or TMC207, PZA, RPE and CFZ were also shown to be more active than current standard regimen of RIF, INH and PZA in murine model of TB [354, 383].

Inclusion of bedaquiline in multidrug regimens for MDR-TB patients typically containing OFX, KAN, PZA, EMB and CS or TZD resulted in culture conversion in 48% patients compared to only 9% in control group [384]. Similarly, addition of bedaquiline during the first 8 weeks to a background regimen significantly reduced the time to culture conversion over 24 weeks and reduced the development of resistance to companion drugs [385]. These studies have shown that addition of bedaquiline to MDR-TB regimens accelerates sputum culture negativity and prevents acquired resistance to companion drugs and may reduce the treatment duration to 12 months from the current 18-24 months. The drug has recently been granted approval on the basis of phase II efficacy and safety data by Food and Drug Administration of the USA for treatment of MDR-TB patients, becoming the first new TB drug in nearly four decades. However, the drug is associated with QT prolongation and an increased risk of death. Consequently, its use is presently limited to those MDR-TB patients who cannot be effectively treated with sufficient number of currently available drugs. A phase III trial to evaluate its efficacy in sputum smear-positive MDR-TB patients is also likely to start soon [386].

Nitroimidazoles are structurally related to metronidazole that has been used extensively to treat human infections by protozoa and anaerobic bacteria. Metronidazole is known to have only modest activity against *M. tuberculosis*. More potent derivatives (PA-824 and delamanid or OPC-67683) of metronidazole have been synthesized recently [387]. These drugs are active against drug-susceptible and drug-resistant *M. tuberculosis* strains indicating a novel mechanism of action. They are active against both, replicating and hypoxic, non-replicating *M. tuberculosis* suggesting their potential in shortening treatment duration. These pro-drugs require nitroreductive activation by a common mechanism involving deazaflavin-dependent glucose 6-phosphate dehydrogenase (Rv0407) and deazaflavin-dependent nitroreductase (Rv3547, Ddn) [388-390].

PA-824, a nitroimidazo-oxazine derivative, developed by TB Alliance, shows potent activity against drug sensitive and drug-resistant (including MDR) strains of *M. tuberculosis* with MIC ranging from 0.06-0.53 mg/L (Table 8.1). No cross-resistance is observed with other first-line drugs indicating a novel mechanism of action and its activity under anaerobic conditions is comparable to RIF [387]. The drug was well tolerated as single, oral dose of 200 mg or higher for up to 14 days but the activity in sputum-positive pulmonary TB patients was nearly same at different doses. However, 800 mg or higher doses resulted in higher creatinine levels in blood [391, 392]. The drug exhibited time-dependent bactericidal action against actively replicating organisms due to inhibition of synthesis of ketomycolates, an essential component of cell wall of tubercle bacilli while poisoning of the respiratory apparatus (cytochrome c oxidase) by nitrous oxide generated during bioreductive activation killed dormant bacilli under anaerobic (hypoxic) conditions [393, 394].

In murine model of TB, PA-824 (100 mg/kg) was as effective as INH (25 mg/kg) in combination therapy with RIF and PZA during initial phase and exhibited better activity than INH or MFX (100 mg/kg) and equivalent to the combination of RIF/INH in the 4 months continuation phase [395]. The combination of PA-824, MFX and PZA in a 6 month regimen was more effective than RIF, INH and PZA regimen, however, addition of PA-824 to RIF, MFX and PZA regimen was unable to shorten the treatment duration from 4 to 3 months [396]. A 3 or 4 drug combination of new agents containing bedaquiline, PA-824 and PNU-100480 and/or CFZ showed superior activity than first-line regimen of RIF, INH and PZA [354]. These studies also showed, for the first time, that a regimen without RIF and INH can cure TB more effectively than the standard first-line regimen and also showed synergy between PA-824 and PZA. In humans, 14-day bactericidal activity of different combinations of PA-824, TMC207, PZA, and MFX in patients with drug-susceptible pulmonary TB showed that PA-824-MFX-PZA or PA-824-PZA combinations were significantly higher than that of bedaquiline-PZA or bedaquiline-PA-824 and comparable with that of standard first-line treatment. These preliminary data have shown that PA-824-MFX-PZA combination is potentially suitable for treating both, drug-susceptible TB and MDR-TB [397, 398]. In murine model of TB, novel 3-drug combinations composed of TMC207, PZA, PA-824, MFX, and RPE cured 100% of treated mice in 2 months while 4 months of first-line regimen including RIF, INH and PZA did not cure any mice. These results reveal novel regimens with potential to shorten the duration of treatment for both drug-susceptible and drug-resistant TB (including MDR-TB) [399]. Phase II clinical trials to assess the mycobactericidal activity, safety and tolerability of PA-824 in different regimens for the treatment of patients with drug-susceptible and MDR pulmonary TB are currently being carried out [400, 401].

Delamanid or OPC67683, a nitro-dihydro-imidazo-oxazole derivative, was developed by Otsuka Pharmaceutical Co. Ltd. to enhance the potency and lower the toxicity of PA-824. Delamanid is structurally related to PA-824 and also requires bioreductive activation by deazaflavin-dependent nitroreductase and inhibits methoxy-mycolic and keto-mycolic acid biosynthesis in *M. tuberculosis* [387, 402]. However, it is more potent against drug sensitive and drug-resistant (including MDR) strains of *M. tuberculosis* with MIC ranging from 0.006-0.024 mg/L (Table 8.1) which is nearly 10 times lower than the MIC of PA-824 [402]. Like PA-824, delamanid is also active against non-replicating persistent *M. tuberculosis* and its activity at 0.1 mg/L is equivalent to RIF at 3 mg/L against intracellular bacilli in macrophages [402]. Cross-resistance between delamanid and PA-824 occurs frequently as both of these drugs are activated by a common mechanism and the resistance is mainly conferred by mutations in *ddn* gene, however, no cross-resistance or antagonism is observed with other first-line drugs. Also, delamanid is not a substrate for human CYP450 enzymes minimizing the potential for adverse drug-drug interactions [388, 402]. In murine models of TB, delamanid was as effective in reducing the bacterial burden as RIF or INH and combination of delamanid, RIF and PZA resulted in much more rapid clearance of bacteria from lung tissue than the standard regimen of RIF, INH, PZA and EMB [402].

Daily oral doses of 100 to 400 mg were well tolerated for 14 days in smear-positive pulmonary TB patients, however, its maximal serum concentration at a dose of 200 mg reached only 0.22 mg/L, which is nearly 8 times lower than for PA-824. Thus delamanid has a MIC 10 times lower than that of PA-824, however, its bioavailability also appears to be nearly 8 times lower than that of PA-824. Similar to the results with PA-824, the EBA values were also nearly equivalent for the entire range of delamanid doses. However, 200 mg and 300 mg doses produced slightly better response in higher frequency of pulmonary TB patients [403]. Delamanid has completed phase II clinical trials for the treatment of patients infected with MDR strains of *M. tuberculosis* and results of few studies have recently been published. Addition of delamanid at a daily dose of 100 mg twice daily or 200 mg twice daily to a background drug regimen developed according to WHO guidelines for the treatment of patients with pulmonary MDR-TB was associated with rapid sputum-culture conversion at 2 months compared to placebo group (45.4% versus 29.6%). The results with the higher doses of delamanid were also similar and most adverse events were mild to moderate in severity and distributed across both, delamanid and placebo groups [404]. Another study that interrogated the duration of delamanid therapy has reported better prognosis among MDR-TB patients who received delamanid ≥6 months, compared to MDR-TB patients who received delamanid for ≤2 months and treatment benefits were also seen among patients with XDR-TB [405]. These findings suggest that treatment with delamanid for 6 months in combination with a WHO optimized background regimen can improve treatment outcome and reduce mortality among patients with both, MDR-TB and XDR-TB [391, 392]. A phase III multicenter, randomized, double blind, placebo controlled trial to evaluate the safety and efficacy of delamanid administered orally as 200 mg daily for 6 months in patients with sputum culture-positive MDR-TB is currently being carried out [406].

New ethylenediamines are derivatives of EMB that have been developed recently. SQ109, a member of this class developed by Sequella Inc., is active against EMB-resistant *M. tuberculosis* strains implying a different mechanism of action [407]. It is active against drug-susceptible and drug-resistant TB including MDR-TB strains with MIC ranging from 0.7 to 1.6 mg/L (Table 8.1) and shows synergistic interaction with INH and RIF as well as with bedaquiline (TMC207) [408, 409]. SQ109, similar to EMB, also inhibits cell wall synthesis in *M. tuberculosis* but inhibits MmpL3, a membrane transporter of trehalose monophosphate while EMB inhibits arabinosyltransferases [134, 410]. In murine model of TB, SQ109 at 25 mg/kg was more effective than

EMB at 100 mg/kg in reducing the bacterial burden, the tissue drug levels were ~10 fold higher than its MIC and substitution of SQ109 for EMB improved the efficacy of first-line combination therapy after 4 and 8 weeks of treatment [407, 408]. In humans, oral doses of SQ109 up to 300 mg are safe and well tolerated with good tissue distribution. The drug has also been combined with several other (TMC207, PA-824 and PNU-100480) experimental drugs for activity against intracellular *M. tuberculosis* and combinations of PNU-100480, TMC207 and SQ109 were fully additive and comparable to standard TB therapy with first-line drugs [409, 411, 412]. SQ109 is currently being evaluated in phase II trials in adults with smear-positive pulmonary TB for extended EBA, safety, tolerability and pharmacokinetic evaluations [413].

More potent oxazolidinone derivaties have been synthesized recently to improve the modest activity of LZD against *M. tuberculosis* and to overcome the problem of toxicity (myelosuppression, neurotoxicity and gastrointestinal disturbance) associated with its extended (>28 days) use for the treatment of MDR-TB/XDR-TB patients [414]. PNU-100480, being developed by Pfizer, is a close structural analog of LZD but is nearly 3 times more active against drug-susceptible and drug-resistant *M. tuberculosis* strains with MIC range of 0.03 to 0.5 mg/L (Table 8.1) [415]. In murine model of TB, PNU-100480 activity was comparable to INH and its inclusion in various combinations improved the EBA of first-line therapy during early stage of treatment [416, 417]. Combination therapy with PNU-100480, MFX and PZA or bedaquiline, PA-824 and PNU-100480 was more active than standard first-line therapy with RIF, INH and PZA suggesting that new combinations with novel agents have the potential to shorten treatment duration for both, drug-susceptible and drug-resistant TB [354, 416]. Combinations of PNU-100480, TMC207, and SQ109 are fully additive and are predicted to have cumulative activity comparable to the current standard first-line TB therapy [411]. Phase I studies on safety, tolerability and pharmacokinetics of PNU-100480 have recently been completed. Drug doses of 100, 300 or 600 mg twice daily or 1200 mg once daily up to 14 days or 600 mg twice daily for 28 days were well tolerated and did not produce any significant adverse drug reactions in healthy volunteers [418]. The drug exhibits synergistic interactions with PZA, bedaquiline (TMC207) and SQ109 [409, 411, 412] and is currently in phase II clinical trials.

Another new oxazolidinone derivative (AZD5847), developed by Astra-Zeneca, is also bactericidal against drug-susceptible and drug-resistant strains of *M. tuberculosis* [414]. Generally much less is known about AZD5847 than for PNU-100480. Its MIC_{90} for drug-resistant *M. tuberculosis* isolates was reported as 1 mg/L. The *in vitro* generated drug-resistant mutants show point mutations in *rrl* encoding 23S rRNA and *rplC* encoding the L3 subunit of the 50S ribosomal subunit. In murine intracellular infection model of TB, AZD5847 exhibited superior bactericidal activity compared to LZD. The drug is also active against rapidly dividing and slowly dividing *M. tuberculosis* based on studies in high-dose and low-dose aerosol infection models. Two phase I studies to assess the safety, tolerability and pharmacokinetics of single and multiple ascending oral doses of AZD5847 over 14-day period have been completed recently [419, 420]. The drug was well tolerated and the bioavailability of AZD5847 was better with food intake but decreased with increasing doses in fasted individuals. The estimated human oral dose for AZD5847 is 500 mg twice daily. Other investigational doses of AZD5847 (800 mg twice daily and 1200 mg once daily) are currently being evaluated in phase II trials for EBA (0-14 days) during treatment of uncomplicated fully susceptible smear-positive pulmonary TB [421].

Another promising new drug is FAS 20013 (developed by FASgen Inc.). FAS 20013 belongs to the class of β-sulphonylcarboxamides. With an MIC of ~0.8 mg/L (Table 8.1), FAS 20013 is a potent drug against *M. tuberculosis* including MDR-TB strains. The target of FAS 20013 is mycolic acid/cell wall synthesis and the drug appears to kill *M. tuberculosis* more rapidly than the current first-line anti-TB drugs. FASgen Inc. has listed this project on its website (http://www.fasgen.com/pubs-fr.html) (accessed on February 7, 2013 by S. Ahmad). The drug is available orally which makes it suitable for multidrug combination therapy for TB. Also the drug is non-toxic to mammalian cells in cell cultures and is effective against actively dividing intracellular and extracellular tubercle bacilli as well as non-replicating bacilli in anaerobic environment suggesting that it possesses sterilizing activity similar to other first-line drugs RIF and PZA. The drug is also effective against intracellular tubercle bacilli (*M. tuberculosis*-infected macrophages). Furthermore, cross-resistance of FAS 20013 to other first-line drugs is not reported, suggesting the potential of this novel drug for the treatment of both drug-susceptible TB and MDR-TB/XDR-TB and for shortening the treatment duration of current therapy regimens for pulmonary TB.

A pyrrole derivative (LL-3858) is being developed by Lupin India Ltd. however, very limited information about this antimycobacterial agent or its metabolic target is currently vailable. The drug has potent antimycobacterial activity with MIC range of 0.06-0.5 mg/L (Table 8.1) against standard, drug-susceptible and drug-resistant *M. tuberculosis* strains. Pyrrole derivative LL-

3858 showed higher bactericidal activity than INH when administered as monotherapy to infected mice and enhanced the efficacy of first-line therapy with RIF, INH and PZA. Pyrrole LL3858 is currently in phase I clinical trials [295, 332].

8B.2. New Drugs in Preclinical Development

Several new and potent anti-TB drugs have also been developed recently that show activity against both, drug-susceptible and drug-resistant *M. tuberculosis* strains and are in various stages of preclinical development. Some of these important new agents are also listed in Table 8.1 and are described below.

A new class of sulfur containing heterocyclic nitro-benzothiazinone derivatives (BTZ) have been developed that show potent activity against *M. tuberculosis.* The BTZ043 is the most active compound in the series and inhibits synthesis of cell wall arabinans that are essential for maintaining cell wall integrity in mycobacteria. Depletion of arabinans results in cell lysis and bacterial death [422]. With MIC of 0.001-0.004 mg/L, BTZ043 showed ~20 times more potent bactericidal activity than INH against *M. tuberculosis.* It is active against MDR-TB and XDR-TB strains implying a novel mechanism of action [423]. Like INH, BTZ043 is mainly active against actively dividing organisms while its activity against non-replicating, metabolically inert tubercle bacilli is markedly less, suggesting that BTZ043 blocks a critical step in active metabolism of *M. tuberculosis* [422]. The drug was active in a mouse infection model causing reduction in bacterial burden in lungs and spleen of infected animals [422]. BTZ043 (a pro-drug) contains a benzene ring and a reactive nitro group that requires reductive activation leading to a nitroso derivative. The drug acts as a suicide inhibitor as it is activated by an FAD-dependent decaprenylphosphoryl-β-d-ribofuranose 2'-oxidase (DprE1 encoded by *rv3790*) involved in cell-wall biogenesis and the activated form of BTZ043 then binds covalently to an active site residue (Cys387) of DprE1 to form a stable semimercaptal [422-426]. This action blocks the conversion of decaprenylphosphoryl-β-D-ribose to decaprenylphosphoryl-β- D-arabinofuranose, a precursor for the synthesis of cell wall arabinan. The BTZ043-resistant *M. tuberculosis* strains contain mutations at *dprE1* codon 387 (Cys387Ser or Cys387Gly) and mutant DprE1 enzymes reduce the drug to inert metabolites [424-426]. Drug-interaction profiles of BTZ043 with several approved or experimental anti-TB drugs (including RIF, INH, EMB, MFX,

MEP-CLV, TMC207, PA-824 and SQ-109) showed additive or synergistic interactions while no antagonism was found between BTZ043 and the tested compounds [427]. The drug is now ready for clinical trials.

The N-(2-(4-methoxyphenoxy) ethyl)-3,5-dinitrobenzamide (DNB1), a dinitrobenzamide derivative, is structurally related to benzothiazinones as it also contains a benzene ring with a nitro group attached at position 3. DNB1 also requires activation by DprE1 and the activated form subsequently inhibits decaprenylphosphoryl-β- D-arabinofuranose synthesis by blocking DprE1. This action blocks the synthesis of both, lipoarabinomannan and arabinogalactan, major components of mycobacterial cell wall. DNB1 showed potent activity against drug-susceptible and XDR-TB strains as it inhibited replication of *M. tuberculosis* inside macrophages [428]. DNB1 exhibits cross-resistance with BTZ043 as both drugs target DprE1, however, it appears to be more potent (MIC of <0.001 mg/L) than BTZ043 [428, 429]. The drug also exhibits lower cell toxicity and is currently under further clinical development.

During solid phase synthesis and screening of a focused library of diamines by phenotypic cell-based assays during the development of SQ109, several new dipiperidine analogues including SQ609 were also found to be active against *M. tuberculosis* [430]. SQ609 at 4 mg/L inhibited intracellular growth of *M. tuberculosis* inside macrophages without showing any detectable toxicity and once daily dosing at 10 mg/kg was effective in preventing weight loss and prolonging therapeutic effects of treatment in murine model of TB [431]. SQ609 likely inhibits cell wall biosynthesis in *M. tuberculosis* and is currently under further clinical development.

Another compound (SQ641) developed recently, is an analogue of capuramycin, a naturally occurring nucleoside-based antibiotic produced by *Streptomyces griseus* that targets phospho-*N*-acetylmuramyl-pentapeptide translocase 1 (TL1), an essential enzyme involved in the biosynthesis of bacterial cell walls [432]. TL1 is an attractive target for antibacterial therapy as inhibition of TL1 activity leads to bacterial cell death and the absence of this activity in mammalian cells reduces the toxicity concerns. SQ641 was selected from a library of >7,000 capuramycin analogues created at Daiichi-Sankyo in Japan that showed good activity against *M. tuberculosis* and other mycobacteria [433]. SQ641 with an MIC of 1 mg/L kills *M. tuberculosis* faster than first-line drugs, INH and RIF. The drug is also active against MDR-TB strains and shows synergistic activity with INH, EMB, SM and experimental ethylenediamine derivative, SQ109 [432]. Due to poor solubility in water and poor intracellular activity, SQ641 was recently dissolved in α-tocopheryl polyethylene glycol 1000 succinate (TPGS), a water-soluble vitamin E analogue or incorporated into TPGS-micelles. The drug at a dose of 25 mg/kg, administered intravenously twice per week in a mouse model of TB, significantly reduced bacterial burden in the lungs [433]. Other analogues of SQ641 have also been synthesized to improve water solubility and some of these compounds have shown improved intracellular killing of *M. tuberculosis* in murine macrophages [434]. Sequella Inc. is currently carrying out further clinical development of SQ641.

Another nucleoside antibiotic, caprazamycin, produced by *Streptomyces* sp. MK730-62F2, was first isolated at Microbial Chemistry Research Foundation in Japan and belongs to the 6'-N-alkyl-5'-beta-O-aminoribosyl-glycyluridine class of antibiotics. Other analogues of caprazamycin were also synthesized that showed more potent antibacterial activity. CPZEN-45, a water soluble compound, is a semi-synthetic analogue of caprazamycin that has shown potential as an effective anti-TB agent [435]. CPZEN-45 is active, *in vitro,* against both, replicating and non-replicating (dormant) bacilli suggesting that it may have potential in shortening the duration of treatment. CPZEN-45 shows an MIC range of 1.6-6.2 mg/L (Table 8.1) against drug-susceptible and MDR *M. tuberculosis* strains. In murine model of TB, CPZEN-45 was effective in reducing bacterial burden during infection with drug-susceptible and XDR *M. tuberculosis* strains. Lilly TB Drug Discovery Initiative is carrying out further development of CPZEN-45 [436].

DC-159a is a new, fourth-generation 8-methoxy FQ bearing a 3-aminopyrrolidyl substitution that is active (MIC range of 0.03 to 1.0 mg/L, Table 8.1) against drug-susceptible and some FQ-resistant MDR *M. tuberculosis* strains. The activity of DC-159a was 4-32-fold higher than other currently available quinolones including MFX [437]. Importantly, DC-159a exhibited bactericidal activity against FQ-resistant *M. tuberculosis* strains containing A90V and/or D94G substitution(s) in GyrA while G88C mutation in GyrA conferred resistance to DC-159a [438]. A G88C and D94H double mutation in *gyrA* gene was recently shown to confer high-level resistance to DC-159a in *in vitro* generated resistant strains [438]. Thus, DC-159a may remain active against some FQ-resistant MDR-TB strains as well as some XDR-TB strains with common *gyrA* mutations. In murine model of TB, DC-159a exhibited dose-dependent bactericidal activity, which was superior to MFX in both, initial and continuation phases of treatment [439]. Further studies incorporating DC-159a in various drug combinations containing new and existing drugs are currently being carried out for shortening the duration of drug-susceptible TB and for the effective treatment of some FQ-resistant MDR-TB and XDR-TB patients.

8B.3. Promising Lead Compounds as Anti-TB Drugs

Several promising lead compounds have also been synthesized recently. 1,5-Diarylpyrrole derivative, [1, 5-diaryl-2-methyl-3-(4-methylpiperazin-1-yl)methyl-pyrrole], designated as BM212 has shown potent activity against both, drug-susceptible and drug-resistant *M. tuberculosis* strains including intracellular bacilli residing in macrophages [440]. Other analogues of BM212 containing the same 1,5-diarylpyrrole scaffold have also been synthesized more recently that exhibited even better activity than BM212 with MIC values comparable to first-line drugs INH, RIF and SM and low cytotoxicity [441-443]. The cellular target of these anti-TB drugs has now been identified as MmpL3 (mycobacterial membrane protein, large), a putative membrane transporter of mycolic acids, by isolation and analysis of *in vitro* generated drug-resistant strains [444]. Conditional gene expression studies have shown that MmpL3 is an essential protein for mycobacterial growth and is invloved in the translocation of trehalose monomycolates across the plasma membrane during synthesis of cell wall arabinogalactan or in the formation of virulence-associated, trehalose-containing glycolipids in the outer membrane. Other inhibitors of MmpL3 have also been synthesized that abolish translocation of mycolic acids from the cytoplasm to the periplasmic side of the plasma membrane and show potent bactericidal activity against *M. tuberculosis* [445].

Pyridomycin, a naturally occurring antibiotic produced by *Streptomyces pyridomyceticus* or *Dactylosporangium fulvum,* shows specific activity (MIC of 0.31-0.63 mg/L) against various mycobacteria including *M. tuberculosis* with little detectable activity against other Gram-positive and Gram-negative bacteria [446, 447]. However, its mechanism of action against tubercle bacilli remained unknown and its potential as an anti-TB drug was not properly assessed. A recent study has shown that pyridomycin has bactericidal activity against *M. tuberculosis* growing extracellularly and inside macrophages. Strikingly, the intracellular killing activity of pyridomycin was superior to INH and comparable to RIF, however, the drug also exhibited considerable cytotoxicity and was not effective against non-replicating dormant bacilli [448]. Pyridomycin, like INH, also targets NADH-dependent enoyl ACP reductase (encoded by *inhA*) and an *in vitro* generated pyridomycin-resistant *M. tuberculosis* strain contained D148G mutation located near the NADH binding pocket in *inhA* [449]. However, unlike INH, pyridomycin is an active drug and binds differently to InhA as the pyridomycin-resistant *M. tuberculosis* strain remained susceptible to INH [448]. Since INH is a prodrug and 50-95% of INH-resistant strains contain mutations in *katG* gene, pyridomycin is effective against most INH-resistant clinical *M. tuberculosis* strains [448]. Thus, pyridomycin serves as an attractive compound for the synthesis of more effective and less toxic derivatives for further evaluation.

Several other compounds are also in lead identification and optimization stage of discovery and only few of these are briefly described. Compound 5, a quinoxaline 1,4-di-oxide derivative has been synthesized with activity against drug-susceptible, polydrug-resistant and MDR *M. tuberculosis* isolates, suggesting a novel mechanism of action. It exhibited bactericidal activity against both, actively dividing and non-replicating persistent tubercle bacilli in a murine model of TB [450]. Similar to PA-824, Compound 5 is also a prodrug that is also activated by bioreductive mechanism, however, the activation mechanism is different than used by PA-824 since Compound 5 remained active on all PA-824-resistant *M. tuberculosis* strains. Quinolone-isoxazole hybrid compounds have also been synthesized and Compound 7g (a quinoline-isoxazole derivative) also showed bactericidal activities against actively dividing and non-replicating persistent tubercle bacilli [451]. Two novel methylbenzothiazole-based compounds (notably Compound 7j) and three novel tetrahydroindazole-based compounds (notably Compound 6a) have also been synthesized recently and showed potent (MIC of <2 μM) activity against actively dividing *M. tuberculosis* in vitro with no detectable cytotoxicity [452, 453].

Synthesis of deoxy-sugar derivatives have identified, 2,3-dideoxy hex-2-anopyranosid-4-uloses as promising new anti-TB drugs. Compound 5g was particularly more potent with MIC range of 0.78-1.56 mg/L against drug-susceptible and MDR *M. tuberculosis* strains and also exhibited activity against intracellular tubercle bacilli [454]. Other compounds such as indeno[2,1-c]quinolines, 1,4-diarylpiperazines, benzo[j]phenanthridine-7,12-diones, 1,2,4-oxadiazoles, heterocyclic oxazolidinones (such as RBx 8700) and mefloquine-oxazolidine derivatives have been synthesized and exhibit potent activity against drug-susceptible and MDR *M. tuberculosis* isolates including intracellularly growing bacilli [455-460]. These drugs add to the new drugs that are already in various stages of clinical and preclinical development for the treatment and proper management of MDR-TB and XDR-TB patients.

Chapter IX

Concluding Remarks

The global TB epidemic continues to be a great public health challenge. TB mainly afflicts the economically weaker sections of society in both, developed and developing countries. Lack of resources for national TB control programs in developing countries resulted in poor case detection and cure rates, particularly in high TB incidence countries. The inadequate/ inappropriate therapy due to inability of poor patients to pay for drugs, poor quality of anti-TB drugs and non-adherence to treatment (regimen and duration) resulted in the evolution of drug-resistant *M. tuberculosis* strains. Today, drug-resistant TB and MDR-TB have become prevalent in many parts of the world and XDR-TB strains are emerging rapidly.

Most of the diagnostic methods used currently in resource-poor settings were developed several decades ago. New diagnostic methods are urgently needed to identify the spectrum of *M. tuberculosis* infections (including latent infection, active disease and drug-resistant TB). Rapid nucleic acid-based tests for drug-resistant TB are an encouraging development. Though still expensive, the line probe assays and Xpert MTB/RIF for rapid diagnosis of TB and RIF resistance in pulmonary specimens are well advanced for routine use but still cannot replace standard diagnostic methods such as clinical/radiological assessment and culture and conventional DST. More work is needed for TB diagnosis in extrapulmonary specimens, in HIV-coinfected patients and children. Development of technologies suitable for poor patients in resource-poor settings should be the priority. Point of care tests using untreated sputum, blood or urine with simple equipment will be of immense benefit in the future. The recent success with global AIDS effort has shown that much can be accomplished when effective diagnostic and treatment procedures are matched with appropriate funding and political will.

Current therapeutic agents are old and inadequate to meet the challenge. There are few safe and effective drugs to treat drug-resistant TB in HIV-coinfected patients. Successful eradication of TB requires new drugs and new drug regimens. There have been some advancements in TB drug development pipeline during the last few years. Currently, 6 compounds, some affecting new targets, are in late stages of clinical development. New compounds must be carefully assessed in controlled clinical trials of combination regimens that will be suitable for economically weaker patients in resource-limited settings and should be effective in HIV/TB coinfected patients.

References

[1] Daniel, TM. The history of tuberculosis. *Respir Med* 2006, 100, 1862-1870.

[2] Cole, ST; Brosch, R; Parkhill, J; Garnier, T; Churcher, C; Harris, D; Gordon, SV; Eigelmeir, K; Gas, S; Barry, CE III; Tekaia, F; Badcock, K; Basham, D; Brown, D; Chillingworth, T; Conner, R; Davies, R; Devlin, K; Feltwell, T; Genties, S; Hamlin, N; Holroyd, S; Hornsby, T; Jagels, K; Krogh, A; McLean, J; Moule, S; Murphy, L; Oliver, K; Osborne, J; Quuail, MA; Ranjanderam, MA; Rogers, J; Rutter, S; Seeger, K; Skelton, J; Squares, R; Squares, S; Sulston, JE; Taylor, K; Whitehead, S; Barrell, BG. Deciphering the biology of *Mycobacterium tuberculosis* from the complete genome sequence. *Nature* 1998, 393, 537-544.

[3] Garnier, T; Eiglmeier, K; Camus, JC; Medina, N; Mansoor, H; Pryor, M; Duthoy, S; Grondin, S; Lacroix, C. Monsempe, C; Simon, S; Harris, B; Atkin, R; Doggett, J; Mayes, R; Keating, L; Wheeler, PR; Parkhill, J; Barrell, BG; Cole, ST; Gordon, SV; Hewinson, RG. The complete genome sequence of *Mycobacterium bovis*. *Proc Natl Acad Sci USA* 2003, 100, 7877-7882.

[4] Pawlowski, A; Jansson, M; Skold, M; Rottenberg, M. E.; Kallenius, G. Tuberculosis and HIV co-infection. *PLoS Pathog* 2012, 8, article no. e1002464.

[5] Wright, A; Zignol, M; Van Deun, A; Falzon D, Gerdes SR, Feldman K, Hoffner S, Drobniewski F, Barrera L, van Soolingen D, Boulabhal F, Paramasivan CN, Kam KM, Mitarai S, Nunn P, Raviglione M; Global Project on Anti-Tuberculosis Drug Resistance Surveillance for the

Global Project on Anti-Tuberculosis Drug Resistance Surveillance. Epidemiology of antituberculosis drug resistance 2002-2007: an updated analysis of the Global Project on Anti-Tuberculosis Drug Resistance Surveillance. *Lancet* 2009, 373,1861-1873.

[6] World Health Organization, "Multidrug and extensively drug-resistant TB (M/XDR-TB): 2010 global report on surveillance and response," *WHO/HTM/TB/2010.3*, Geneva, Switzerland: WHO, 2010.

[7] Frieden, TR; Sterling, TR; Munsiff, SS; Watt, CJ; Dye, C. Tuberculosis. *Lancet* 2003, 362, 887-899.

[8] Dooley, K; Chaisson, RE. Tuberculosis and diabetes mellitus: convergence of two epidemics. *Lancet Infect Dis* 2009, 9, 737-746.

[9] Harries, AD; Lin, Y; Satyanarayana, S; Lonnroth, K; Li, L; Wilson, N; Chauhan, LS; Zachariah, R; Baker, MA; Jeon, CY; Murray, MB; Maher, D; Bybgbjerg, IC; Enarson, DA; Billo, NE; Kapur, A. The looming epidemic of diabetes-associated tuberculosis: learning lessons from HIV-associated tuberculosis. *Int J Tuberc Lung Dis* 2011, 15, 1436-1444.

[10] Janbaz, KH; Qadir, MI; Ahmad, B; Sarwar, A; Yaqoob, N; Masood, MI. Tuberculosis-burning issues: multidrug resistance and HIV-coinfection. *Crit Rev Microbiol* 2012, 38, 267-275.

[11] Dye, C; Williams, BG. The population dynamics and control of tuberculosis. *Science* 2010, 328, 856-861.

[12] Ahmad, S. Pathogenesis, immunology and diagnosis of latent *Mycobacterium tuberculosis* infection. *Clin Develop Immunol* 2011, 2011, Article ID 814943.

[13] Cooper, AM. Cell-mediated immune responses in tuberculosis. *Annu Rev Immunol* 2009, 27, 393-422.

[14] Barry, CE III; Boshoff HI; Dartois, V; Dick, T.; Ehrt, S; Flynn, J; Schnappinger, D; Wilkinson, RJ; Young, D. The spectrum of latent tuberculosis: rethinking the biology and intervention strategies. *Nat Rev Microbiol* 2009, 7, 845-855.

[15] Davis, JM; Ramakrishnan, L. The role of the granuloma in expansion and dissemination of early tuberculous infection. *Cell* 2009, 136, 37-49.

[16] Ahmad, S. New approaches in the diagnosis and treatment of latent tuberculosis infection. *Resp Res* 2010, 11, article no. 169.

[17] Young, DB; Gideon, HP, Wilkinson, RJ. Eliminating latent tuberculosis. *Trends Microbiol* 2009, 17, 193-198.

[18] Rustad, TR; Sherrid, AM; Minch, KJ; Sherman, DR. Hypoxia: a window into *Mycobacterium tuberculosis* latency. *Cell Microbiol* 2009, 11, 1151-1159.

[19] Gupta, A; Kaul, A; Tsolaki, AG; Kishore, U; Bhakta, S. *Mycobacterium tuberculosis*: immune evasion, latency and reactivation. *Immunobiology*, 2012, 217, 363-374.

[20] Ottenhoff, TH; Kaufmann, SH. Vaccines against tuberculosis: where are we and where do we need to go? *PLoS Pathog* 2012, 8, Article no. e1002607.

[21] World Health Organization, "Global tuberculosis report 2012," WHO report 2012. *WHO/HTM/TB/2008.393*. Geneva, Switzerland: WHO, 2012.

[22] Zignol, M; van Gemert, W; Falzon, D; Sismanidis, C; Glaziou, P; Floyd, K; Raviglione, M. Surveillance of anti-tuberculosis drug resistance in the world: an updated analysis, 2007-2010. *Bull World Health Organ* 2012, 90, 111-119D.

[23] Palomino, JC; Martin, A; Von Groll, A; Portaels, F. Rapid culture-based methods for drug-resistance detection in *Mycobacterium tuberculosis*. *J Microbiol Meth* 2008, 75, 161-166.

[24] World Health Organization, "Anti-tuberculosis drug resistance in the world: fourth Global report," *WHO/HTM/TB/2008.394*. Geneva, Switzerland: WHO, 2008.

[25] Zhao, Y; Xu, S; Wang, L; Chin, DP; Wang, S; Jiang, G; Xia, H; Zhou, Y; Li, Q; Ou, X; Pang, Y; Song, Y; Zhao, B; Zhang, H; He, G; Guo, J; Wang, Y. National survey of drug-resistant tuberculosis in China. *N Engl J Med* 2012, 366, 2161-2170.

[26] Michael, JS; John, TJ. Extensively drug-resistant tuberculosis in India: a review. *Indian J Med Res* 2012, 136, 599-604.

[27] Dheda, K; Migliori, GB. The global rise of extensively drug-resistant tuberculosis: is the time to bring back sanatoria now overdue? *Lancet* 2012, 379, 773-775.

[28] Skrahina, A; Hurevich, H; Zalutskaya, A; Sahalchyk, E; Astrauko, A; van Gemert, W; Hoffner, S; Rusovich, V; Zignol, M. Alarming levels of drug-resistant tuberculosis in Belarus: results of a survey in Minsk. *Eur Respir J* 2012, 39, 1425-1431.

[29] Migliori, GB; Loddenkemper, R; Blasi, F; Raviglione, MC. 125 years after Robert Koch's discovery of the tubercle bacillus: the new XDR-TB threat. Is "science" enough to tackle the epidemic? *Eur Respir J* 2007, 29, 423-427.

[30] Velayati, AA; Masjedi, MR; Farnia, P; Tabarsi, P; Ghanavi, J; ZiaZarifi, AH. Emergence of new forms of totally drug-resistant tuberculosis bacilli: super extensively drug-resistant tuberculosis or totally drug resistant strains in Iran. *Chest* 2009, 136, 420-425.

[31] Shah, NS; Richardson, J; Moodley, P; Moodley, S; Babaria, P; Ramtahal, M. Increasing drug resistance in extensively drug-resistant tuberculosis, South Africa. *Emerg Infect Dis* 2011, 17, 510-513.

[32] Udwadia, ZF; Amale, RA; Ajbani, KK; Rodriguez, C. Totally drug-resistant tuberculosis in India. *Clin Infect Dis* 2012, 54, 579-581.

[33] Velayati, AA; Farnia, P; Masjedi, MR; Ibrahim, TA; Tabarsi, P; Haroun, RZ; Kuan, HO; Ghanavi, J; Farnia, P; Varahram, M. Totally drug-resistant tuberculosis strains: evidence of adaptation at the cellular level. *Eur Respir J* 2009, 34, 1202-1203.

[34] Kim, SJ. Drug-susceptibility testing in tuberculosis: methods and reliability of results. *Eur Respir J* 2005, 25, 564-569.

[35] Cegielski, P; Nunn, P; Kurbatova, EV; Weyer, K; Dalton, TL; Wares, DF; Iademarco, MF; Castro, KG; Raviglione, M. Challenges and controversies in defining totally drug-resistant tuberculosis. *Emerg Infect Dis* 2012, 18, article no. e2.

[36] Orenstein, EW; Basu, S; Shah, NS; Andrews, JR; Friedland, GH; Moll, AP; Gandhi, NR; Galvani, AP. Treatment outcomes among patients with multidrug-resistant tuberculosis: systematic review and meta-analysis. *Lancet Infect Dis* 2009, 9, 153-161.

[37] Ahmad, S; Mokaddas, E. Recent advances in the diagnosis and treatment of multidrug-resistant tuberculosis. *Respir Med* 2009, 103, 1777-1790.

[38] Ahmad, S; Mokaddas, E. New approaches in the diagnosis and treatment of susceptible, multidrug-resistant and extensively drug-resistant tuberculosis. *Kuwait Med J* 2012, 44, 3-19.

[39] Mitnick, CD; Shin, SS; Seung, KJ; Rich, ML; Atwood, SS; Furin, JJ; Fitzmaurice, GM; Alcantara Viru, FA; Appleton, SC; Bayona, JN; Bonilla, CA; Chalco, K; Choi, S; Franke, MF; Fraser, HS; Guerra, D; Hurtado, RM; Jazayeri, D; Joseph, K; Llaro, K; Mestanza, L; Mukherjee, JS; Muñoz, M; Palacios, E; Sanchez, E; Sloutsky, A; Becerra, MC. Comprehensive treatment of extensively drug-resistant tuberculosis. *N Engl J Med* 2008, 359, 563-574.

[40] Jacobson, KR; Tierney, DB; Jeon, CY; Mitnick, CD; Murray, MB. Treatment outcomes among patients with extensively drug-resistant

tuberculosis: systematic review and meta-analysis. *Clin Infect Dis* 2010, 51, 6-14.

[41] Gandhi, NR; Andrews, JR; Burst, JCM; Montreuil, M; Weissman, D; Heo M; Moll, AP; Friedland GH; Shah, NS. Risk factors for mortality among MDR- and XDR-TB patients in a high HIV prevalence setting. *Int J Tuberc Lung Dis* 2012, 16, 90-97.

[42] Medical Research Council. Streptomycin treatment of pulmonary tuberculosis: a Medical Research Council Investigation. *Br Med J* 1948, 2, 769-782.

[43] Mitchison, DA. Role of individual drugs in the chemotherapy of tuberculosis. *Int J Tuberc Lung Dis* 2000, 4, 796-806.

[44] Blumberg HM, Burman WJ, Chaisson RE, Daley CL, Etkind SC, Friedman LN, et al. American Thoracic Society; CDC; Infectious Disease Society of America. Treatment of tuberculosis. *Am J Respir Crit Care Med* 2003, 167, 603-662.

[45] Mitchison, D; Davies, G. The chemotherapy of tuberculosis: past, present and future. *Int J Tuberc Lung Dis* 2012, 16, 724-732.

[46] Raviglione, MC; Pio, A. Evolution of WHO policies for tuberculosis control, 1948-2001. *Lancet* 2002, 359, 775-780.

[47] Frieden, TR; Munsiff, SS. The DOTS strategy for controlling the global tuberculosis epidemic. *Clin Chest Med* 2005, 26, 197-205.

[48] World Health Organization, "Treatment of tuberculosis: guidelines for national programmes 4th ed.," *WHO/HTM/TB/2009.420*, Geneva, Switzerland: WHO, 2009.

[49] Yee, D; Valiquette, C; Pelletier, M; Parisien, I; Rocher, I; Menzies, D. Incidence of serious side effects from first-line antituberculosis drugs among patients treated for active tuberculosis. *Am J Respir Crit Care Med* 2003, 167, 1472-1477.

[50] Wells, CD; Cegielski, JP; Nelson, LJ; Laserson, KF; Holtz TH; Finlay, A; Castro, KG; Weyer, K. HIV infection and multidrug-resistant tuberculosis-the perfect storm. *J Infect Dis* 2007, 196 (Suppl 1), S86-S107.

[51] Manosuthi, W; Sungkanuparph, S; Tantanathip, P; Lueangniyomkul, A; Mankatitham, W; Prasithsirskul, W; Burapatarawong, S; Thongyen, S; Likanonsakul, S; Thawornwa, U; Prommool, V; Ruxrungtham, K; N2R Study Team. A randomized trial comparing plasma drug concentrations and efficacies between 2 nonnucleoside reverse transcriptase inhibitor-based regimens in HIV-infected patients receiving rifampicin: the N2R study. *Clin Infect Dis* 2009, 48, 1752-1759.

[52] Kwara, A; Ramachandran, G; Swaminathan, S. Dose adjustment of the non-nucleoside reverse transcriptase inhibitors during concurrent rifampicin-containing tuberculosis therapy: one size does not fit all. *Expert Opin Drug Metab Toxicol* 2010, 6, 55-68.

[53] Zhang, J; Zhu, L; Stonier, M; Coumbis, J; Xu, X; Wu, Y; Arikan, D; Farajallah, A; Bertz, R. Determination of rifabutin dosing regimen when administered in combination with ritonavir-boosted atazanavir. *J Antimicrob Chemother* 2011, 66, 2075-2082.

[54] Jiménez-Corona, ME; Cruz-Hervert, LP; García-García, L; Ferreyra-Reyes, L; Delgado-Sánchez, G; Bobadilla-Del-Valle, M; Canizales-Quintero, S; Ferreira-Guerrero, E; Báez-Saldaña, R; Téllez-Vázquez, N; Montero-Campos, R; Mongua-Rodriguez, N; Martínez-Gamboa, RA; Sifuentes-Osornio, J; Ponce-de-León, A. Association of diabetes and tuberculosis: impact on treatment and post-treatment outcomes. *Thorax* 2013, 68, 214-220.

[55] David, HL. Probability distribution of drug resistant mutants in unselected populations of *Mycobacterium tuberculosis*. *Appl Microbiol* 1970, 20, 810-814.

[56] Kempker, RR; Rabin, AS; Nikolaishvili, K; Kalandadze, I; Gogishvili, S; Blumberg, HM; Vashakidze, S. Additional drug resistance in *Mycobacterium tuberculosis* isolates from resected cavities among patients with multidrug-resistant or extensively drug-resistant pulmonary tuberculosis. *Clin Infect Dis* 2012, 54, e51-e54.

[57] Boulanger, C; Hollender, E; Farrell, K; Stambaugh, JJ; Maasen, D; Ashkin, D; Symes, S; Espinoza, LA; Rivero, RO; Graham, JJ; Peloquin, CA. Pharmakokinetic evaluation of rifabutin in combination with lopinavir-ritonavir in patients with HIV infection and active tuberculosis. *Clin Infect Dis* 2009, 49, 1305-1311.

[58] Mitchison, DA. Pharmacokinetic/pharmacodynamic parameters and the choice of high-dosage rifamycins. *Int J Tuberc Lung Dis* 2012, 16, 1186-1189.

[59] Maus, CE; Pilkaytis, BB; Shinnick, TM. Molecular analysis of cross-resistance to capreomycin, kanamycin, amikacin and viomycin in *Mycobacterium tuberculosis*. *Antimicrob Agents Chemother* 2005, 49, 3192-3197.

[60] Georghiou, SB; Magana, M; Garfein, RS; Catanzaro, DG; Catanzaro, A; Rodwell, TC. Evaluation of genetic mutations associated with *Mycobacterium tuberculosis* resistance to amikacin, kanamycin and

capreomycin: a systematic review. *PLoS One* 2012, 7, article no. e33275.

[61] Johnson, JL; Hadad, DJ; Boom, WH; Daley, CL; Peloquin, CA; Eisenach, KD; Jankus, DD; Debanne, SM; Charlebois, ED; Maciel, E; Palaci, M; Dietze, R. Early and extended early bactericidal activity of levofloxacin, gatifloxacin and moxifloxacin in pulmonary tuberculosis. *Int J Tuberc Lung Dis* 2006, 10, 605-612.

[62] Ahmad, S; Mokaddas, E. Role of fluoroquinolones in the treatment of tuberculosis. *Rev Health Care* 2012, 3, 19-33.

[63] Burman, WJ; Goldberg, S; Johnson, JL; Muzanye, G; Engle, M; Mosher, AW; Choudhri, S; Daley, CL; Munsiff, SS; Zhao, Z; Vernon, A; Chaisson, RE. Moxifloxacin versus ethambutol in the first two months of treatment for pulmonary tuberculosis. Moxifloxacin versus ethambutol in the first two months of treatment for pulmonary tuberculosis. *Am J Respir Crit Care Med* 2006, 174, 331-338.

[64] Rustomjee, R; Lienhardt, C; Kanyok, T; Davies, GR; Levin, J; Mthiyane, T; Reddy, C; Sturm, AW; Sirgel, FA; Allen, J; Coleman, DJ; Fourie, B; Mitchison, DA; Gatifloxacin for TB (OFLOTUB) study team. A phase II study of the sterilizing activities of ofloxacin, gatifloxacin and moxifloxacin in pulmonary tuberculosis. *Int J Tuberc Lung Dis* 2008, 12, 128-138.

[65] Dorman, SE; Johnson, JL; Goldberg, S; Muzanye, G; Padayatchi, N; Bozeman, L; Heilig, CM; Bernardo, J; Choudhri, S; Grosset, JH; Guy, E; Guyadeen, P; Leus, MC; Maltas, G; Menzies, D; Nuermberger, EL; Villarino, M; Vernon, A; Chaisson, RE; Tuberculosis Trials Consortium. Substitution of moxifloxacin for isoniazid during intensive phase treatment for pulmonary tuberculosis. *Am J Respir Crit Care Med* 2009, 180, 273-280.

[66] Conde, MB; Efron, A; Loredo, C; De Souza, GR; Graça, NP; Cezar, MC; Ram, M; Chaudhary, MA; Bishai, WR; Kritski, AL; Chaisson, RE. Moxifloxacin versus ethambutol in the initial treatment of tuberculosis: a double-blind, randomized, controlled phase II trial. *Lancet* 2009, 373, 1183-1189.

[67] Chiang, C-Y; Schaaf, HS. Management of drug-resistant tuberculosis. *Int J Tuberc Lung Dis* 2010, 14, 672-682.

[68] Ahmad, S; Mokaddas, E. New challenges in the treatment of tuberculosis in the 21st century. *Treat Strat Resp* 2011, 1, 100-110.

[69] World Health Organization, "Treatment of tuberculosis: guidelines for national programmes," *WHO/CDS/TB/2008.108 (revised)*. Geneva, Switzerland: WHO, 2008.

[70] Dooley, KE; Obuku, EA; Durakovic, N; Belitsky, V; Mitnick, C; Nuermberger, EL; on behalf of the Efficacy Subgroup, RESIST-TB. World Health Organization Group 5 Drugs for the Treatment of Drug-Resistant Tuberculosis: Unclear Efficacy or Untapped Potential? *J Infect Dis* 2013, 207, 1352-1358.

[71] Xu, H-B; Jiang, R-H; Li, L; Xiao, H-P. Linezolid in the treatement of MDR-TB: a retrospective clinical study. *Int J Tuberc Lung Dis* 2012, 16, 358-363.

[72] Cox, H; Ford, N. Linezolid for the treatment of complicated drug-resistant tuberculosis: a systematic review and meta-analysis. *Int J Tuberc Lung Dis* 2012, 16, 447-454.

[73] Mainardi, JL; Hugonnet, JE; Gutmann, L; Arthur, M. Fighting resistant tuberculosis with old compounds: the carbapenem paradigm. *Clin Microbiol Infect* 2011, 17, 1755-1756.

[74] Gonzalo, X; Drobniewski, F. Is there a place for β-lactams in the treatment of multidrug-resistant/extensively drug-resistant tuberculosis? Synergy between meropenem and amoxicillin/clavulanate. J Antimicrob Chemother 2013, 68, 366-369.

[75] Centers for Disease Control and Prevention. Extensively drug-resistant tuberculosis-United States, 1993-2006. *MMWR Morb Mortal Wkly Rep* 2007, 56, 250-253.

[76] Andini, N; Nash, KA. Intrinsic macrolide resistance of the Mycobacterium tuberculosis complex is inducible. *Antimicrob Agents Chemother* 2006, 50, 2560-2562.

[77] Stoffels, K; Traore, H; Vanderbist, F; Fauville-Dufaux, M. The effect of combined tobramycin-clarithromycin on *Mycobacterium tuberculosis* isolates. *Int J Tuberc Lung Dis* 2009, 13, 1041-1044.

[78] Ramaswamy, S; Musser, JM. Molecular genetics basis of antimicrobial agent resistance in *Mycobacterium tuberculosis*: 1998 update. *Tuberc Lung Dis* 1998, 79, 3-29.

[79] Zhang, Y; Yew, WW. Mechanisms of drug resistance in *Mycobacterium tuberculosis*. *Int J Tuberc Lung Dis* 2009, 13, 1320-1330.

[80] Almeida Da Silva, PE; Palomino, JC. Molecular basis and mechanisms of drug resistance in *Mycobacterium tuberculosis*: classical and new drugs. *J Antimicrob Chemother* 2011, 66, 1417-1430.

[81] Sandgren, A; Strong, M; Muthukrishnan, P; Weiner, BK; Church, GM; Murray, MB. Tuberculosis drug resistance mutation database. *PLoS Med* 2009, 6, article no. e2.

[82] Zhang, Y; Heym, B; Allen, B; Young, D; Cole, ST. The catalase-peroxidase gene and isoniazid resistance of *Mycobacterium tuberculosis*. *Nature* 1992, 358, 591-593.

[83] Heym, B; Alzari, PM; Honore, N; Cole, ST. Missense mutations in the catalase-peroxidase gene, *kat*G, are associated with isoniazid resistance in *Mycobacterium tuberculosis*. *Mol Microbiol* 1995, 15, 235-245.

[84] Donald, PR; Diacon, AH. The early bactericidal activity of anti-tuberculosis drugs: a literature review. *Tuberculosis (Edinburgh)* 2008, 88(Suppl 1), S75-S83.

[85] Larsen, MH; Vilcheze, C; Kremer, L; Besra, GS; Parsons, L; Salfinger, M; Heifets, L; Hazbon, MH; Alland, D; Sacchettini, JC; Jacobs, WR Jr. Overexpression of *inhA*, but not *kasA*, confers resistance to isoniazid and ethionamide in *Mycobacterium smegmatis*, *M. bovis* BCG and *M. tuberculosis*. *Mol Microbiol* 2002, 46, 453-466.

[86] Ramaswamy, S; Reich, R; Dou, S; Jasperse, L; Pan, X; Wanger, A; Quituga, T; Graviss, EA. Single nucleotide polymorphisms in genes associated with isoniazid resistance in *Mycobacterium tuberculosis*. *Antimicrob Agents Chemother* 2003, 47, 1241-1250.

[87] Marttila, HJ; Soini, H; Eerola, E; Vyshnevskaya, E; Vyshnevskiy, BI; Otten, TF; Vasilyef, AV; Viljanen, MK. A Ser315Thr substitution in KatG is predominant in genetically heterogeneous multidrug-resistant *Mycobacterium tuberculosis* isolates originating from the St. Petersburg area in Russia. *Antimicrob Agents Chemother* 1998, 42, 2443-2445.

[88] Ahmad, S; Fares, E; Araj, GF; Chugh, TD; Mustafa, AS. Prevalence of S315T mutation within the *katG* gene in isoniazid-resistant clinical *Mycobacterium tuberculosis* isolates from Dubai and Beirut. *Int J Tuberc Lung Dis* 2002, 6, 920-926.

[89] Abal, AT; Ahmad, S; Mokaddas, E. Variations in the occurrence of the S315T mutation within the *katG* gene in isoniazid-resistant clinical *Mycobacterium tuberculosis* isolates from Kuwait. *Microb Drug Resist* 2002, 8, 99-105.

[90] Hazbon, MH; Brimacombe, M; del Valle, MB; Cavatore, M; Guerrero, MI; Verma-Basil, M; Billman-Jacobe, H; Lavender, F; Fyfe, J; Garcia-Garci, L; Leon, CI; Bose, M; Chavez, F; Murray, M; Eisenach, KD; Sifuentes-Osornio, JS; Cave, MD; de Leon, AP; Alland, D. Population genetics study of isoniazid resistance mutations and evolution of

multidrug-resistant *Mycobacterium tuberculosis. Antimicrob Agents Chemother* 2006, 50, 2640-2649.

[91] Guo, H; Seet, Q; Denkin, S; Parsons, L; Zhang, Y. Molecular characterization of isoniazid-resistant clinical isolates of *Mycobacterium tuberculosis* from the USA. *J Med Microbiol* 2006, 55, 1527-1531.

[92] Yao, C; Zhu T, Li Y, Zhang L, Zhang B, Huang J, Fu W. Detection of *rpoB, katG* and *inhA* gene mutations in M*ycobacterium tuberculosis* clinical isolates from Chongqing as determined by microarray. *Clin Microbiol Infect* 2010, 16, 1639-1643.

[93] Ioerger, TR; Koo, S; No, EG; Chen, X; Larsen, MH; Jacobs, WR Jr; Pillay, M; Sturm, AW; Sacchettini, JC. Genome analysis of multi- and extensively-drug-resistant tuberculosis from KwaZulu-Natal, South Africa. *PLoS One* 2009, 4, article no. e7778.

[94] Liu, CH; Li, HM; Lu, N; Wang, Q; Hu, YL; Yang, X; Hu, YF; Woo, PC; Gao, GF; Zhu, B. Genomic sequence based scanning for drug resistance-associated mutations and evolutionary analysis of multidrug-resistant and extensively drug-resistant *Mycobacterium tuberculosis. J Infect* 2012, 65, 412-422.

[95] Casali, N; Nikolayevskyy, V; Balabanova, Y; Ignatyeva, O; Kontsevaya, I; Harris, SR; Bentley, SD; Parkhill, J; Nejentsev, S; Hoffner, SE; Horstmann, RD; Brown, T; Drobniewski, F. Microevolution of extensively drug-resistant tuberculosis in Russia. *Genome Res* 2012, 22, 735-745.

[96] Schmalstieg, AM; Srivastava, S; Belkaya, S; Deshpande, D; Meek, C; Leff, R; van Oers, NS; Gumbo, T. The antibiotic resistance arrow of time: efflux pump induction is a general first step in the evolution of mycobacterial drug resistance. *Antimicrob Agents Chemother* 2012, 56, 4806-4815.

[97] Machado, D; Couto, I; Perdigão, J; Rodrigues, L; Portugal, I; Baptista, P; Veigas, B; Amaral, L; Viveiros, M. Contribution of efflux to the emergence of isoniazid and multidrug resistance in *Mycobacterium tuberculosis*. *PLoS One* 2012, 7, article no. e34538.

[98] Wang, XD; Gu, J; Wang, T; Bi, LJ; Zhang, ZP; Cui, ZQ; Wei, HP; Deng, JY; Zhang, XE. Comparative analysis of mycobacterial NADH pyrophosphatase isoforms reveals a novel mechanism for isoniazid and ethionamide inactivation. *Mol Microbiol* 2011, 82, 1375-1391.

[99] Ramos, RM; Perez, JM; Baptista, LA; de Amorim, HL. Interaction of wild type, G68R and L125M isoforms of the arylamine-N-

acetyltransferase from *Mycobacterium tuberculosis* with isoniazid: a computational study on a new possible mechanism of resistance. *J Mol Model* 2012, 18, 4013-4024.

[100] Rosenthal, IM; Zhang, M; Williams, KN; Peloquin, CA; Tyagi, S; Vernon, AA; Bishai, WR; Chaisson, RE; Grosset, JH; Nuermberger, EL. Daily dosing of rifapentine cures tuberculosis in three months or less in the murine model. *PLoS Med* 2007, 4, article no. e344.

[101] Telenti, A; Imboden, P; Marchesi, F; Lowrie, D; Cole, S; Colston, MJ; Matter, L; Schopfer, K; Bodmer, T. Detection of rifampicin-resistance mutations in *Mycobacterium tuberculosis. Lancet* 1993, 341, 647-650.

[102] Nolan, CM; Williams, DL; Donald Cave, M; Eisenach, KD; El-Hajj, H; Hooton, TM; Thompson, RL; Goldberg, SV. Evolution of rifampin resistance in human immunodeficiency virus-associated tuberculosis. *Am J Respir Crit Care Med* 1995, 152, 1067-1071.

[103] A. Vernon, W. Burman, D. Benator, A. Khan, and L. Bozeman. Acquired rifamycin monoresistance in patients with HIV-related tuberculosis treated with once-weekly rifapentine and isoniazid. *Lancet* 1999, 353, 1843-1847.

[104] Mokaddas, E; Ahmad, S; Abal, AT; Al-Shami, AS. Molecular fingerprinting reveals familial transmission of rifampin-resistant tuberculosis in Kuwait. *Ann Saudi Med* 2005, 25, 150-153.

[105] Mukinda, FK; Theron, D; van der Spuy, GD; Jacobson, KR; Roscher, M; Streicher, EM; Musekiwa, A; Coetzee, GJ; Victor, TC; Marais, BJ; Nachega, JB; Warren, RM; Schaaf, HS. Rise in rifampicin-monoresistant tuberculosis in Western Cape, South Africa. *Int J Tuberc Lung Dis* 2012, 16, 196-202.

[106] Yuen, LKW; Leslie, D; Coloe, PJ. Bacteriological and molecular analysis of rifampin-resistant *Mycobacterium tuberculosis* strains isolated in Australia. *J Clin Microbiol* 1999, 37, 3844-3850.

[107] Hirano, K; Abe, C; Takahashi, M. Mutations in the *rpoB* gene of rifampin-resistant *Mycobacterium tuberculosis* strains isolated mostly in Asian countries and their rapid detection by line probe assay. *J Clin Microbiol* 1999, 37, 2663-2666.

[108] Ahmad, S; Araj, GF; Akbar, PK; Fares, E; Chugh, TD; Mustafa, AS. Characterization of *rpoB* mutations in rifampin-resistant *Mycobacterium tuberculosis* isolates from the Middle East. *Diagn Microbiol Infect Dis* 2000, 38, 227-232.

[109] Van Rie, A; Warren, R; Mshanga, I; Jordaan, AM; Van Der Spuy, G; Richardson, M; Simpson, J; Gie, RP; Enarson, DA; Beyers, N; Van

Helden, PD; Victor, TC. Analysis for a limited number of gene codons can predict drug resistance of *Mycobacterium tuberculosis* in a high-incidence community. *J Clin Microbiol* 2001, 39, 636-641.

[110] Ahmad, S; Mokaddas, E; Fares, E. Characterization of *rpoB* mutations in rifampin-resistant clinical *Mycobacterium tuberculosis* isolates from Kuwait and Dubai. *Diagn Microbiol Infect Dis* 2002, 44, 245-252.

[111] Siddiqi, N; Shamim, M; Hussain, S; Choudhary, RK; Ahmed, N; Prachee; Banerjee, S; Savithri, GR; Alam, M; Pathak, N; Amin, A; Hanief, M; Katoch, VM; Sharma, SK. Hasnain, SE. Molecular characterization of multidrug-resistant isolates of *Mycobacterium tuberculosis* from patients in North India. *Antimicrob Agents Chemother* 2002, 46, 443-450.

[112] Ma, X; Wang, H; Deng, Y; Liu, Z; Xu, Y; Pan, X; Musser, JM; Graviss, EA. *rpoB* gene mutations and molecular characterization of rifampin-esistant *Mycobacterium tuberculosis* isolates from Shandong Province, China. *J Clin Microbiol* 2006, 44, 3409-3412.

[113] Sheng, J; Li, J; Sheng, G; Yu, H; Huang, H; Cao, H; Lu, Y; Deng, X. Characterization of *rpoB* mutations associated with rifampin resistance in *Mycobacterium tuberculosis* from eastern China. *J Appl Microbiol* 2008, 105, 904-911.

[114] Heep, M; Brandstatter, B; Rieger, U; Lehn, N; Richter, E; Rusch-Gerdes, S; Niemann, S. Frequency of *rpoB* mutations inside and outside the cluster I region in rifampin-resistant clinical *Mycobacterium tuberculosis* isolates. *J Clin Microbiol* 2001, 39, 107-110.

[115] Ahmad, S; Mokaddas, E. The occurrence of rare *rpoB* mutations in rifampicin-resistant *Mycobacterium tuberculosis* isolates from Kuwait. *Int J Antimicrob Agents* 2005, 26, 205-212.

[116] Wang, Q; Yue, J; Zhang, L; Xu, Y; Chen, J; Zhang, M; Zhu, B; Wang, H; Wang, H. A newly identified 191A/C mutation in the Rv2629 gene that was significantly associated with rifampin resistance in *Mycobacterium tuberculosis*. *J Proteome Res* 2007, 6, 4564-4571.

[117] Van Deun, A; Barrera, L; Bastian, I; Fattorini, L; Hoffmann, H; Kam, KM; Rigouts, L; Rüsch-Gerdes, S; Wright, A. *Mycobacterium tuberculosis* strains with highly discordant rifampin susceptibility test results. *J Clin Microbiol* 2009, 47, 3501-3506.

[118] Siu, GK; Zhang, Y; Lau, TC; Lau, RW; Ho, PL; Yew, WW; Tsui, SK; Cheng, VC; Yuen, KY; Yam, WC. Mutations outside the rifampicin resistance-determining region associated with rifampicin resistance in

Mycobacterium tuberculosis. *J Antimicrob Chemother* 2011, 66, 730-733.

[119] Ahmad, S; Al-Mutairi, NM; Mokaddas, E. Variations in the occurrence of specific rpoB mutations in rifampicin-resistant *Mycobacterium tuberculosis* isolates from patients of different ethnic groups in Kuwait. *Indian J Med Res* 2012, 135, 756-762.

[120] Bahrmand, AR; Titov, L; Tasbiti, AH; Yari, S; Graviss, EA. High-level rifampin resistance correlates with multiple mutations in the *rpoB* gene of pulmonary tuberculosis isolates from the Afghanistan border of Iran. *J Clin Microbiol* 2009, 47, 2744-2750.

[121] Cavusoglu, C; Karaca-Derici, Y; Bilgic, A. *In-vitro* activity of rifabutin against rifampicin-esistant *Mycobacterium tuberculosis* isolates with known *rpoB* mutations. *Clin Microbiol Infect* 2004, 10, 662-665.

[122] Yoshida, S; Suzuki, K; Iwamoto, T; Tsuyuguchi, K; Tomita, M; Okada, M; Sakatani, M. Comparison of rifabutin susceptibility and *rpoB* mutations in multidrug-resistant *Mycobacterium tuberculosis* strains by DNA sequencing and the line probe assay. *J Infect Chemother* 2010, 16, 360-363.

[123] Chen, HY; Yu, MC; Huang, WL; Wu, MH; Chang, YL; Che, CR; Jou, R. Molecular detection of rifabutin-susceptible *Mycobacterium tuberculosis*. *J Clin Microbiol* 2012, 50, 2085-2088.

[124] Tan, Y; Hu, Z; Zhao, Y; Cai, X; Luo, C; Zou, C; Liu, X. The beginning of the *rpoB* gene in addition to the rifampin resistance determination region might be needed for identifying rifampin/rifabutin cross-resistance in multidrug-resistant *Mycobacterium tuberculosis* isolates from Southern China. *J Clin Microbiol* 2012, 50, 81-85.

[125] García, AB; Palacios, JJ; Ruiz, MJ; Barluenga, J; Aznar, F; Cabal, MP; García, JM; Díaz, N. Strong in vitro activities of two new rifabutin analogs against multidrug-resistant *Mycobacterium tuberculosis*. *Antimicrob Agents Chemother* 2010, 54, 5363-5365.

[126] Gill, SK; Xu, H; Kirchhoff, PD; Cierpicki, T; Turbiak, AJ; Wan, B; Zhang, N; Peng, KW; Franzblau, SG; Garcia, GA; Showalter, HD. Structure-based design of novel benzoxazinorifamycins with potent binding affinity to wild-type and rifampin-resistant mutant *Mycobacterium tuberculosis* RNA polymerases. *J Med Chem* 2012, 55, 3814-3826.

[127] Comas, I; Borrell, S; Roetzer, A; Rose, G; Malla, B; Kato-Maeda, M; Galagan, J; Niemann, S; Gagneux, S. Whole-genome sequencing of rifampicin-resistant *Mycobacterium tuberculosis* strains identifies

compensatory mutations in RNA polymerase genes. *Nat Genet* 2011, 44, 106-110.

[128] Scorpio, A; Zhang, Y. Mutations in *pncA*, a gene encoding pyrazinamidase/nicotinamidedase, cause resistance to the antituberculous drug pyrazinamide in tubercle bacillus. *Nat Med* 1996, 2, 662-667.

[129] Shi, W; Zhang, X; Jiang, X; Yuan, H; Lee, JS; Barry, CE 3rd; Wang, H; Zhang, W; Zhang, Y. Pyrazinamide inhibits trans-translation in *Mycobacterium tuberculosis*. *Science* 2011, 333, 1630-1632.

[130] Yüksel, P; Tansel, O. Characterization of *pncA* mutations of pyrazinamide-resistant *Mycobacterium tuberculosis* in Turkey. *New Microbiol* 2009, 32, 153-158.

[131] Zhang, H; Bi, LJ; Li, CY; Sun, ZG; Deng, JY; Zhang, XE. Mutations found in the *pncA* gene of *Mycobacterium tuberculosis* in clinical pyrazinamide-resistant isolates from a local region of China. *J Int Med Res* 2009, 37, 1430-1435.

[132] Muthaiah, M; Jagadeesan, S; Ayalusamy, N; Sreenivasan, M; Prabhu, SS; Muthuraj, U; Senthilkumar, K; Veerappan, S. Molecular epidemiological study of pyrazinamide-resistance in clinical isolates of *Mycobacterium tuberculosis* from south India. *Int J Mol Sci* 2010, 11, 2670-2680.

[133] Kim, HJ; Kwak, HK; Lee, J; Yun, YJ; Lee, JS; Lee, MS; Min, SY; Park, SK; Kang, HS; Maeng, YH; Kim, SY; Kim, SY; Kook, YH; Kim, YR; Lee, KH. Patterns of *pncA* mutations in drug-resistant *Mycobacterium tuberculosis* isolated from patients in South Korea. *Int J Tuberc Lung Dis* 2012, 16, 98-103.

[134] Telenti, A; Phillipp, W; Sreevatsan, S; Bernasconi, C; Stockbauer, KE; Wieles, B; Musser, JM; Jacobs, Jr WR. The *emb* operon, a unique gene cluster of *Mycobacterium tuberculosis* involved in resistance to ethambutol. *Nat Med* 1997, 3, 567-570.

[135] Ramaswamy, S; Amin, AG; Koksel, S; Stager, CE; Dou, S-J; El Sahly, H; Moghazeh, SL; Kreiswirth, BN; Musser, JM. Molecular genetic analysis of nucleotide polymorphisms associated with ethambutol resistance in human isolates of *Mycobacterium tuberculosis*. *Antimicrob Agents Chemother* 2000, 44, 326-336.

[136] Parsons, LM; Salfinger, M; Clobridge, A; Dormandy, J; Mirabello, L; Polletta, VL; Sanic, A; Sinyavskiy, O; Larsen, SC; Driscoll, J; Zickas, G; Taber, HW. Phenotypic and molecular characterization of

Mycobacterium tuberculosis isolates resistant to both isoniazid and ethambutol. *Antimicrob Agents Chemother* 2005, 49, 2218-2225.

[137] Mokrousov, I; Ottem, T; Vyshnevskiy, B; Narvskaya, O. Detection of *embB306* mutations in ethambutol-susceptible clinical isolates of *Mycobacterium tuberculosis* from Northwestern Russia: implications for genotypic resistance testing. *J Clin Microbiol* 2002, 40, 3810-3813.

[138] Hazbon, MH; Bobadilla del Valle, M; Guerrero, MI; Varma-Basil, M; Filliol, I; Cavatore, M; Colangeli, R; Safi, H; Billman-Jacobe, H; Lavender, C; Fyfe, J; Garcia-Garcia, L; Davidow, A; Brimacombe, M; Leon, CI; Porras, T; Bose, M; Chaves, F; Eisenach, KD; Sifuentes-Osornio, J; Ponce de Leon, A; Cave, MD; Alland, D. Role of *embB* codon 306 mutations in *Mycobacterium tuberculosis* revisited: a novel association with broad drug resistance and IS*6110* clustering rather than ethambutol resistance. *Antimicrob Agents Chemother* 2005, 49, 3794-3802.

[139] Ahmad, S; Jaber, AA; Mokaddas, E. Frequency of *embB* codon 306 mutations in ethambutol-susceptible and -resistant clinical *Mycobacterium tuberculosis* isolates in Kuwait. *Tuberculosis (Edinburgh)* 2007, 87, 123-129.

[140] Safi, H; Sayers, B; Hazbon, MH; Alland, D. Transfer of *embB* codon 306 mutations into clinical *Mycobacterium tuberculosis* strains alters susceptibility to ethambutol, isoniazid and rifampin. *Antimicrob Agents Chemother* 2008, 52, 2027-2034.

[141] Safi, H; Fleischmann, RD; Peterson SN, Jones MB, Jarrahi B, Alland D. Allelic exchange and mutant selection demonstrate that common clinical *embCAB* gene mutations only modestly increase resistance to ethambutol in *Mycobacterium tuberculosis*. *Antimicrob Agents Chemother* 2010, 54, 103-108.

[142] Plinke, C; Walter, K; Aly, S; Ehlers, S; Niemann, S. *Mycobacterium tuberculosis embB* codon 306 mutations confer moderately increased resistance to ethambutol *in vitro* and *in vivo*. *Antimicrob Agents Chemother* 2011, 55, 2891-2896.

[143] Ahmad, S; Itani, L; Araj, GF; Fares, E. Varying prevalence of *embB* codon 306 mutations in ethambutol-resistant clinical *Mycobacterium tuberculosis* isolates in Beirut and Dubai. *J Chemother* 2008, 20, 285-287.

[144] Starks, AM; Gumusboga, A; Plikaytis, BB; Shinnick, TM; Posey, JE. Mutations at *embB* codon 306 are an important molecular indicator of

ethambutol resistance in *Mycobacterium tuberculosis*. *Antimicrob Agents Chemother* 2009, 53, 1061-1066.

[145] Furin, J. The clinical management of drug-resistant tuberculosis. *Curr Opin Pulm Med* 2007, 13, 212-217.

[146] Sreevatsan, S; Pan, X; Stockbauer, KE; Williams, DL; Kreisworth, BN; Musser, JM. Characterization of *rpsL* and *rrs* mutations in streptomycin-resistant *Mycobacterium tuberculosis* isolates from diverse geographic localities. *Antimicrob Agents Chemother* 1996, 40, 1024-1026.

[147] Tudo, G; Rey, E; Borrell, S; Alcaide, F; Codina, G; Coll, P; Casabona, NM; Montemayar, M; Moure, R; Orcau, A; Salvado, M; Vicente, E; Martin, JG. Characterization of mutations in streptomycin-resistant *Mycobacterium tuberculosis* clinical isolates in the area of Barcelona. *J Antimicrob Chemother* 2010, 65, 2341-2346.

[148] Spies, FS; Ribeiro, AW; Ramos, DF; Ribeiro, MO; Martin, A; Palomino, JC; Rossetti, ML; da Silva, PE; Zaha, A. Streptomycin resistance and lineage-specific polymorphisms in *Mycobacterium tuberculosis gidB* gene. *J Clin Microbiol* 2011, 49, 2625-2630.

[149] Spies, FS; Almeida de Silva, PE; Ribeiro, MO; Rossetti, ML; Zaha, A. Identification of mutations related to streptomycin resistance in clinical isolates of *Mycobacterium tuberculosis* and possible involvement of efflux mechanism. *Antimicrob Agents Chemother* 2008, 52, 2947-2949.

[150] Juréen, P; Angeby, K; Sturegård, E; Chryssanthou, E; Giske, CG; Werngren, J; Nordvall, M; Johansson, A; Kahlmeter, G; Hoffner, S; Schön, T. Wild-type MIC distributions for aminoglycoside and cyclic polypeptide antibiotics used for treatment of *Mycobacterium tuberculosis* infections. *J Clin Microbiol* 2010, 48, 1853-1858.

[151] Maus, CE; Pilkaytis, BB; Shinnick, TM. Mutation of *tlyA* confers capreomycin resistance in *Mycobacterium tuberculosis*. *Antimicrob Agents Chemother* 2005, 49, 571-577.

[152] Johansen, SK; Maus, CE; Plikaytis, BB; Douthwaite, S. Capreomycin binds across the ribosomal subunit interface using tlyA-encoded 2'O-methylation in 16S and 23S rRNAs. *Mol Cell* 2006, 23, 173-182.

[153] Jugheli, L; Bzekalava, N; de Rijk, P; Fisstte, K; Portaels, F; Rigouts, L. High-level cross-resistance between kanamycin, amikacin and capreomycin, among *Mycobacterium tuberculosis* isolates from Georgia and a close relation with mutations in the *rrs* gene. *Antimicrob Agents Chemother* 2009, 53, 5064-5068.

[154] Dalton, T; Cegielski, P; Akksilp, S; Asencios, L; Caoili, JC; Cho, S-N. Prevalence of and risk factors for resistance to second-line drugs in people with multidrug-resistant tuberculosis in eight countries: a prospective cohort study. *Lancet* 2012, 380, 1406-1417.

[155] Zaunbrecher, MA; David Sikes Jr, R; Metchock, B; Shinnick, TM; Posey, JM. Overexpression of the chromosomally encoded aminoglycoside acetyltransferase *eis* confers kanamycin resistance in *Mycobacterium tuberculosis*. *Proc Natl Acad Sci USA* 2009, 106, 20004-20009.

[156] Ginsburg, AS; Grosset, JH; Bishai, WR. Fluoroquinolones, tuberculosis, and resistance. *Lancet Infect Dis* 2003, 3, 432-442.

[157] Moadebi, S; Harder, CK; Fitzgerald, MJ; Elwood, KR; Marra, F. Fluoroquinolones for the treatment of pulmonary tuberculosis. *Drugs* 2007, 67, 2077-2099.

[158] Maruri, F; Sterling, TR; Kaiga, AW; Blackman, A; van der Heijden, YF; Mayer, C; Cambau, E; Aubry, A. A systematic review of gyrase mutations associated with fluoroquinolone-resistant *Mycobacterium tuberculosis* and a proposed gyrase numbering system. *J Antimicrob Chemother* 2012, 67, 819-831.

[159] Escribano, I; Rodriguez, JC; Llorca, B; Garcia-Pachon, E; Ruiz, M; Royo, G. Importance of the efflux pump systems in the resistance of *Mycobacterium tuberculosis* to fluoroquinolones and linezolid. *Chemotherapy* 2007, 53, 397-401.

[160] Takiff, HE; Salazar, L; Guerrero, C; Philipp, W; Huang, WM; Kreiswirth, B; Cole, ST; Jacobs, WR Jr; Telenti, A. Cloning and nucleotide sequence of *Mycobacterium tuberculosis gyrA* and *gyrB* genes and detection of quinolone resistance mutations. *Antimicrob Agents Chemother* 1994, 38, 773-780.

[161] Aubry, A; Veziris, N; Cambau, E; Truffot-Pernot, C; Jarlier, V; Fisher, M. Novel gyrase mutations in quinolone-resistant and hypersusceptible clinical isolates of *Mycobacterium tuberculosis*: functional analysis of mutant enzymes. *Antimicrob Agents Chemother* 2006, 50, 104-112.

[162] Von Groll, A; Martin, A; Jureen, P; Hoffner, S; Vandamme, P; Portaels, F; Palomino, JC; da Silva, PA. Fluoroquinolone resistance in *Mycobacterium tuberculosis* and mutations in *gyrA* and *gyrB*. *Antimicrob Agents Chemother* 2009, 53, 4498-4500.

[163] Malik, S; Willby, M; Sikes, D; Tsodikov, OV; Posey, JE. New insights into fluoroquinolone resistance in *Mycobacterium tuberculosis*:

functional genetic analysis of gyrA and gyrB mutations. *PLoS One*, 2012, 7, article no. e39754.

[164] Wang, JY; Lee, LN; Lai, HC; Wang, SK; Jan, IS; Yu, CJ; Hsueh, PR; Yang, PC. Fluoroquinolone resistance in *Mycobacterium tuberculosis* isolates: associated genetic mutations and relationship to antimicrobial exposure. *J Antimicrob Chemother* 2007, 59, 860-865.

[165] Sirgel, FA; Warren, RM; Streicher, EM; Victor, TC; van Helden, PD; Böttger, EC. gyrA mutations and phenotypic susceptibility levels to ofloxacin and moxifloxacin in clinical isolates of *Mycobacterium tuberculosis*. *J Antimicrob Chemother* 2012, 67, 1088-1093.

[166] Vannelli, TA; Dykman, A; Ortiz de Montellano, PR. The antituberculosis drug ethionamide is activated by a flavoprotein monooxygenase. *J Biol Chem* 2002, 277, 12824-12829.

[167] Fraaije, MW; Kamerbeek, NM; Heidekamp, AJ; Fortin, R; Janssen, DB. The prodrug activator EthA from *Mycobacterium tuberculosis* is a Baeyer-Villger monooxygenase. *J Biol Chem* 2004, 279, 3354-3360.

[168] DeBarber, AE; Mdluli, K; Bosman, M; Bekker, LG;Barry III, CE. Ethionamide activation and sensitivity in multidrug-resistant *Mycobacterium tuberculosis*. *Proc Natl Acad Sci USA* 2000, 97, 9677-9682.

[169] Morlock, GP; Metchock, B; Sikes, D; Crawford, JT; Cooksey, RC. *ethA, inhA*, and *katG* loci of ethionamide-resistant clinical *Mycobacterium tuberculosis* isolates. *Antimicrob Agents Chemother* 2003, 47, 3799-3805.

[170] Vilchèze, C; Av-Gay, Y; Attarian, R; Liu, Z; Hazbón, MH; Colangeli, R; Chen, B; Liu, W; Alland, D; Sacchettini, JC; Jacobs Jr, WR. Mycothiol biosynthesis is essential for ethionamide susceptibility in *Mycobacterium tuberculosis*. *Mol Microbiol* 2008, 69, 1316-1329.

[171] Belardinelli, JM; Morbidoni, HR. Mutations in the essential FAS II β-hydroxyacyl ACP dehydratase complex confer resistance to thiacetazone in *Mycobacterium tuberculosis* and *Mycobacterium kansasii*. *Mol Microbiol* 2012, 86, 568-579.

[172] Feng, Z; Barletta, RG. Roles of *Mycobacterium smegmatis* D-alanine:D-alanine ligase and D-alanine racemase in the mechanisms of action of and resistance to the peptidoglycan inhibitor D-cycloserine. *Antimicrob Agents Chemother* 2003, 47, 283-291.

[173] Chen, JM; Uplekar, S; Gordon, SV; Cole, ST. A point mutation in *cycA* partially contributes to the D-cycloserine resistance trait of

Mycobacterium bovis BCG vaccine strains. *PLoS One* 2012, 7, article no. e43467.

[174] Mathys, V; Wintjens, R; Lefevre, P; Bertout, J; Singhal, A; Kiass, M; Kurepina, N; Wang, XM; Mathema, B; Baulard, A; Kreiswirth, BN; Bifani, P. Molecular genetics of para-aminosalicylic acid resistance in clinical isolates and spontaneous mutants of *Mycobacterium tuberculosis*. *Antimicrob Agents Chemother* 2009, 53, 2100-2109.

[175] Fivian-Hughes, AS; Houghton, J; Davis, EO. *Mycobacterium tuberculosis* thymidylate synthase gene *thyX* is essential and potentially bifunctional, while *thyA* deletion confers resistance to p-aminosalicylic acid. *Microbiology* 2012, 158, 308-318.

[176] Richter, E; Rusch-Gerdes, S; Hillemann, D. First linezolid-resistant clinical isolates of *Mycobacterium tuberculosis. Antimicrob Agents Chemother* 2007, 51, 1534-1536.

[177] Beckert, P; Hillemann, D; Kohl, TA; Kalinowski, J; Richter, E; Niemann, S; Feuerriegel, S. *rplC* T460C identified as a dominant mutation in linezolid-resistant *Mycobacterium tuberculosis* strains. *Antimicrob Agents Chemother* 2012, 56, 2743-2745.

[178] Nyendak, MR; Lewinsohn, DA; Lewinsohn, DM. New diagnostic methods for tuberculosis. *Curr Opin Infect Dis* 2009, 22, 174-182.

[179] Drobniewski, F; Nikolayevskyy, V; Balabanova, Y; Bang, D; Papaventsis, D. Diagnosis of tuberculosis and drug resistance: what can new tools bring us? *Int J Tuberc Lung Dis*. 2012, 16, 860-870.

[180] Palomino, JC. Current developments and future perspectives for TB diagnostics. *Future Microbiol* 2012, 7, 59-71.

[181] Boehme, CC; Nabeta, P; Hillemann, D; Nicol, MP; Shenai, S; Krapp, F; Allen, J; Tahirli, R; Blakemore, R; Rustomjee, R; Milovic, A; Jones, M; O'Brien, SM; Persing, DH; Ruesch-Gerdes, S; Gotuzzo, E; Rodrigues, C; Alland, D; Perkins, MD. Rapid molecular detection of tuberculosis and rifampin resistance. *N Engl J Med* 2010; 363:1005–1015.

[182] Hepple, P; N. Ford, N; McNerney, R. Microscopy compared to culture for the diagnosis of tuberculosis in induced sputum sampllles: a systematic review. *Int J Tuberc Lung Dis* 2012, 16, 579-588.

[183] Brodie, D; Schluger, NW. The diagnosis of tuberculosis. *Clin Chest Med* 2005, 26, 247-271.

[184] Koh, WJ; Ko, Y; Kim, CK; Park, KS; Lee, NY. Rapid diagnosis of tuberculosis and multidrug resistance using a MGIT 960 system. *Ann Lab Med* 2012, 32, 264-269.

[185] Somoskovi, A; Song, Q; Mester, J; Tanner, C; Hale, YM; Parsons, LM; Salfinger M. Use of molecular methods to identify *Mycobacterium tuberculosis* complex (MTBC) and other mycobacterial species and to detect rifampin resistance in MTBC isolates following growth detection with the BACTEC MGIT 960 system. *J Clin Microbiol* 2003, 41, 2822-2826.

[186] Tortoli, E; Mariottini, A; Mazzarelli, G. Evaluation of INNO-LiPA MYCOBACTERIA v2: improved reverse hybridization multiple DNA probe assay for mycobacterial identification. *J Clin Microbiol* 2003, 41, 4418-4420.

[187] Mokaddas, E; Ahmad, S. Species spectrum of nontuberculous mycobacteria isolated from clinical specimens in Kuwait. *Curr Microbiol* 2008, 56, 413-417.

[188] Daley, P; Petrich, A; May, K; Luinstra, K; Rutherford, C; Chedore, P; Jamieson, F; Smieja, M. Comparison of in-house and commercial 16S rRNA sequencing with high-performance liquid chromatograpgy and genotype AS and CM for identification of nontuberculous mycobacteria. *Diagn Microbiol Infect Dis* 2008, 61, 284-293.

[189] Cheng, VC; Yew, WW; Yuen, KY. Molecular diagnostics in tuberculosis. *Eur J Clin Microbiol Infect Dis* 2005, 24, 711-720.

[190] Saleeb, PG; Drake, SK; Murray, PR; Zelazny, AM. Identification of mycobacteria in solid-culture media by matrix-assisted laser desorption ionization-time of flight mass spectrometry. *J Clin Microbiol* 2011, 49, 1790-1794.

[191] El Khéchine, A; Couderc, C; Flaudrops, C; Raoult, D; Drancourt, M. Matrix-assisted laser desorption/ionization time-of-flight mass spectrometry identification of mycobacteria in routine clinical practice. *PLoS One* 2011, 6, article no. e24720.

[192] Hofmann-Thiel, S; Turaev, L; Alnour, T; Drath, L; Mullerova, M; Hoffmann, H. Multi-centre evaluation of the speed-oligo Mycobacteria assay for differentiation of *Mycobacterium spp.* in clinical isolates. *BMC Infect Dis* 2011, 11, article no. 353.

[193] Said, HM; Ismail, N; Osman, A; Velsman, C; Hoosen, AA. Evaluation of TBc identification immunochromatographic assay for rapid identification of *Mycobacterium tuberculosis* complex in samples from broth cultures. *J Clin Microbiol* 2011, 49, 1939-1942.

[194] Roberts, SA; Lowe, O; Pandey, S; Williamson, DA; Newton, S; Vaughan, R. Comparison of the MGIT TBc immunochromatographic assay with the Accuprobe Gen-Probe TB assay for identification of

Mycobacterium tuberculosis complex: results from a low-burden tuberculosis setting. *Diagn Microbiol Infect Dis* 2012, 74, 415-416.

[195] Causse, M; Ruiz, P; Gutierrez-Aroca, JB; Casal, M. Comparison of two molecular methods for rapid diagnosis of extrapulmonary tuberculosis. *J Clin Microbiol* 2011, 49, 3065-3067.

[196] Scott, LE; McCarthy, K; Gous, N; Nduna, M; Van Rie, A; Sanne, I; Venter, WF; Duse, A; Stevens, W. Comparison of Xpert MTB/RIF with other nucleic acid technologies for diagnosing pulmonary tuberculosis in a high HIV prevalence setting: a prospective study. *PLoS Med* 2011, 8, article no. e1001061.

[197] Teo, J; Jureen, R; Chiang, D; Chan, D; Lin, R. Comparison of two nucleic acid amplification assays, the Xpert MTB/RIF assay and the Amplified Mycobacterium Tuberculosis Direct assay, for detection of *Mycobacterium tuberculosis* in respiratory and nonrespiratory specimens. J Clin Microbiol 2011, 49, 3659-3662.

[198] Wang, J; Lee L; Hsu, H; Hsueh, P; Luh, K. Performance assessment of the DR. MTBC screen assay and the BD ProbeTec ET system for direct detection of *Mycobacterium tuberculosis* in respiratory specimens. J Clin Microbiol 2006, 44, 716-719.

[199] Helb, D; Jones, M; Story, E; Boehme, C; Wallace, E; Ho, K; Kop, J; Owens, MR; Rodgers, R; Banada, P; Safi, H; Blakemore, R; Ngoc Lan, NT; Jones-Lopez, EC; Levi, M; Burdy, M; Ayakaka, I; Mugerwa, RD; McMillan, B; Winn-Deen, E; Christel, L; Dailey, P; Perkins, B; Persing, DH; Alland, D. Rapid detection of *Mycobacterium tuberculosis* and rifampin resistance by use of on-demand, near-patient technology. *J Clin Microbiol* 2010, 48, 229–237.

[200] Hillemann, D; Rüsch-Gerdes, S; Boehme, C; Richter, E. Rapid molecular detection of extrapulmonary tuberculosis by the automated GeneXpert MTB/RIF system. *J Clin Microbiol* 2011, 49, 1202-1205.

[201] Malbruny, B; Le Marrec, G; Courageux, K; Leclercq, R; Cattoir, V. Rapid and efficient detection of *Mycobacterium tuberculosis* in respiratory and non-respiratory samples. *Int J Tuberc Lung Dis* 2011, 15, 553-555.

[202] Hanif, SN; Eldeen, HS; Ahmad, S; Mokaddas, E. GeneXpert MTB/RIF for rapid detection of *Mycobacterium tuberculosis* in pulmonary and extra-pulmonary samples. *Int J Tuberc Lung Dis* 2011, 15, 1274-1275.

[203] Armand, S; Vanhuls, P; Delcroix, G; Courcol, R; Lamaitre, N. Comparison of the Xpert MTB/RIF test with an IS6110-TaqMan real-time PCR assay for direct detection of *Mycobacterium tuberculosis* in

respiratory and non-respiratory specimens. *J Clin Microbiol* 2011, 49, 1772-1776.

[204] Chang, K; Lu, W; Wang, J; Zhang, K; Jia, S; Li, F; Deng, S; Chen, M. Rapid and effective diagnosis of tuberculosis and rifampicin resistance with Xpert MTB/RIF assay: a meta-analysis. *J Infect* 2012, 64, 580-588.

[205] Van Rie, A; Mellet, K; John, MA; Scott, L; Page-Shipp, L; Dansey, H; Victor, T; Warren, R. False-positive rifampicin resistance on Xpert® MTB/RIF: case report and clinical implications. *Int J Tuberc Lung Dis* 2012, 16, 206-208.

[206] Kim, SY; Kim, H; Kim, SY; Ra, EK; Joo, SI; Shin, S; Seong, MW; Yoo, CG; Kim, EC; Park, SS. The Xpert® MTB/RIF assay evaluation in South Korea, a country with an intermediate tuberculosis burden. *Int J Tuberc Lung Dis* 2012, 16, 1471-1476.

[207] Meyer-Rath, G; Schnippel, K; Long, L; MacLeod, W; Sanne, I; Stevens, W; Pillay, S; Pillay, Y; Rosen, S. The impact and cost of scaling up GeneXpert MTB/RIF in South Africa. *PLoS One* 2012, 7, article no. e36966.

[208] Bottger, EC. The ins and outs of *Mycobacterium tuberculosis* drug susceptibility testing. *Clin Microbiol Infect* 2011, 17, 1128-1134.

[209] World Health Organization. Policy guidance on TB drug susceptibility testing (DST) of second-line drugs (SLD). Geneva, Switzerland: WHO, 2008. http://www.who.int/tb/features_archive/xdr_mdr_policy_guidance/en. WHO, 2008.

[210] Lin, SG; Desmond, E; Bonato, D; Gross, W; Siddiqi, S. Multicenter evaluation of Bactec MGIT 960 system for second-line drug susceptibility testing of *Mycobacterium tuberculosis* complex. *J Clin Microbiol* 2009, 47, 3630-3634.

[211] Espasa, M; Salvadó, M; Vicente, E; Tudó, G; Alcaide, F; Coll, P; Martin-Casabona, N; Torra, M; Fontanals, D; González-Martín, J. Evaluation of the VersaTREK System Compared to the Bactec MGIT 960 System for First-Line Drug Susceptibility Testing of *Mycobacterium tuberculosis*. *J Clin Microbiol* 2012, 50, 488-491.

[212] Siddiqi, S; Ahmed, A; Asif, S; Behera, D; Javaid, M; Jani, J; Jyoti, A; Mahatre, R; Mahto, D; Richter, E; Rodrigues, C; Visalakshi, P; Rüsch-Gerdes, S. Direct drug susceptibility testing of *Mycobacterium tuberculosis* for rapid detection of multidrug resistance using the Bactec

MGIT 960 system: a multicenter study. *J Clin Microbiol* 2012, 50, 435-440.

[213] Palomino, JC. Newer diagnostics for tuberculosis and multidrug-resistant tuberculosis. *Curr Opin Pulm Med* 2006; 12, 172-178.

[214] Palomino, JC; Martin, A; Portaels, F. Rapid drug resistance detection in *Mycobacterium tuberculosis*. a review of colourimetric methods. *Clin Microbiol Infect* 2007, 13, 754-762.

[215] Bwanga, F; Hoffner, S; Haile, M; Joloba, ML. Direct susceptibility testing for multidrug-resistant tuberculosis: a meta-analysis. *BMC Infect Dis* 2009, 9, article no. 67.

[216] Moore, DA; Shah, NS. Alternative methods of diagnosing drug resistance, what can they do for me? *J Infect Dis* 2011, 204 (Suppl 4), S1110-S1119.

[217] Moore, DA; Evans, CA; Gilman, RH; Caviedes, L; Coronel, J; Vivar, A; Sanchez, E; Piñedo, Y; Saravia, JC; Salazar, C; Oberhelman, R; Hollm-Delgado, MG; LaChira, D; Escombe, AR; Friedland, JS. Microscopic-observation drug-susceptibility assay for the diagnosis of TB. *New Engl J Med* 2006, 355, 1539-1550.

[218] Minion, J; Leung, E; Menzies, D; Pai, M. Microscopic-observation drug susceptibility and thin layer agar assays for the detection of drug resistant tuberculosis: a systematic review and meta-analysis. *Lancet Infect Dis* 2010, 10, 688-698.

[219] Coronel, J; Roper M; Mitchell, S; Castillo, E; Gamarra, N; Drobniewski, F; Luna, G; Mendoza, A; Moore, DA. MODS accreditation process for regional reference laboratories in Peru: validation by GenoType® MTBDRplus. *Int J Tuberc Lung Dis* 2010, 14, 1475-1480.

[220] Shah, NS; Moodley, P; Babaria, P; Moodley, S; Ramtahal, M; Richardson, J; Heysell, S; Li, X; Moll, A; Friedland, G; Sturm, AW; Gandhi, NR. Rapid diagnosis of tuberculosis and multidrug resistance by the microscopic-observation drug-susceptibility assay. *Am J Respir Crit Care Med* 2011, 183, 1427-1433.

[221] Bwanga, F; Haile, M; Joloba, ML; Ochom, E; Hoffner, S. Direct nitrate reductase assay versus microscopic observation drug susceptibility test for rapid detection of MDR-TB in Uganda. *PLoS One* 2011, 6, article no. e19565.

[222] Martin, A; Paasch, F; Von Groll, A; Fissette, K; Almeida, P; Varaine, F; Portaels, F; Palomino, JC. Thin-layer agar for detection of resistance

to rifampincin, ofloxacin and kanamycin in *Mycobacterium tuberculosis*. *Int J Tuberc Lung Dis* 2009, 13, 1301-1304.

[223] Toit, K; Mitchell, S; Balabanova, Y; Evans, CA; Kummik, T; Nikolayevskyy, V; Drobniewski, F. The Colour Test for drug susceptibility testing of *Mycobacterium tuberculosis* strains. *Int J Tuberc Lung Dis* 2012, 16, 1113-1118.

[224] Bwanga, F; Joloba, ML; Haile, M; Hoffner, S. Evaluation of seven tests for the rapid detection of multidrug-resistant tuberculosis in Uganda. *Int J Tuberc Lung Dis* 2010, 14, 890-895.

[225] Ramos, E; Fissette, K; de Rijk, P; Palomino, JC; Martin, A. Integrated detection of multi- and extensively drug-resistant tuberculosis using the nitrate reductase assay. *Int J Tuberc Lung Dis* 2012, 16, 110-113.

[226] Dixit, P; Singh, U; Sharma, P; Jain, A. Evaluation of nitrate reduction assay, resazurin microtiter assay and microscopic observation drug susceptibility assay for first line antitubercular drug susceptibility testing of clinical isolates of *M. tuberculosis*. *J Microbiol Methods*. 2012, 88, 122-126.

[227] Martin, A; Portaels, F; Palomino, JC. Colorimetric redox-indicator methods for the rapid detection of multidrug resistance in *Mycobacterium tuberculosis*: a systematic review and meta-analysis. *J Antimicrob Chemother* 2007, 59, 175-183.

[228] Martin, A; Paasch, F; Docx, S; Fissette, K; Imperiale, B; Ribón, W; González, LA; Werngren, J; Engström, A; Skenders, G; Juréen, P; Hoffner, S; Del Portillo, P; Morcillo, N; Palomino, JC. Multicentre laboratory validation of the colorimetric redox indicator (CRI) assay for the rapid detection of extensively drug-resistant (XDR) *Mycobacterium tuberculosis*. *J Antimicrob Chemother* 2011, 66, 827-833.

[229] Da Silva, PA; Boffo, MMS; de Mattos, IG; Silva, ABS; Palomino, JC; Martin, A; Takiff, HE. Comparison of redox and D29 phage methods for detection of isoniazid and rifampicin resistance in *Mycobacterium tuberculosis*. *Clin Microbiol Infect* 2006, 12, 293-296.

[230] Minion, J; Pai, M. Bacteriophage assays for rifampicin resistance detection in *Mycobacterium tuberculosis*: updated meta-analysis. *Int J Tuberc Lung Dis* 2010, 14, 941-951.

[231] Rondón, L; Piuri, M; Jacobs, WR Jr; de Waard, J; Hatfull, GF; Takiff, HE. Evaluation of fluoromycobacteriophages for detecting drug resistance in *Mycobacterium tuberculosis*. *J Clin Microbiol* 2011, 49, 1838-1842.

[232] World health Organization. The Global Plan to Stop TB 2011-2015. WHO/HTM/STB/20102. Geneva, Switzerland: WHO, 2010.

[233] Dorman, SE. New diagnostic tests for tuberculosis: bench, bedside and beyond. *Clin Infect Dis* 2010, 50 (Suppl. 3), S173-S177.

[234] Tukvadze, N; Kempker, RR; Kalandadze, I; Kurbatova, E; Leonard, MK; Apsindzelashvili, R; Bablishvili, N; Kipiani, M; Blumberg, HM. Use of a molecular diagnostic test in AFB smear positive tuberculosis suspects greatly reduces time to detection of multidrug resistant tuberculosis. *PLoS One* 2012, 7, article no. e31563.

[235] Ahmad, S; Mokaddas, E. Contribution of AGC to ACC and other mutations at codon 315 of the *katG* gene in isoniazid-resistant *Mycobacterium tuberculosis* isolates from the Middle East. *Int J Antimicrob Agents* 2004, 23, 473-479.

[236] Ahmad, S; Mokaddas, E; Jaber, AA. Rapid detection of ethambutol-resistant *Mycobacterium tuberculosis* strains by PCR-RFLP targeting *embB* codons 306 and 497 and *iniA* codon 501 mutations. *Mol Cell Probes* 2004, 18, 299-306.

[237] Caws, M; Tho, DQ; Duy, PM; Lan, NT; Hoa, DV; Torok ME; Chau, TT; Chau, NV; Chinh, NT; Farrar, J. PCR- restriction fragment length polymorphism for rapid, low-cost identification of isoniazid-resistant *Mycobacterium tuberculosis*. *J Clin Microbiol* 2007, 45, 1789-1793.

[238] Mokrousov, I; Otten, T; Filipenko, M; Vyazovaya, A; Chrapov, E; Limeschenko, E; Steklova, L; Vyshnevskiy, B; Narvskaya, O. Detection of isoniazid-resistant *Mycobacterium tuberculosis* strains by a multiplex allele-specific PCR assay targeting *katG* codon 315 variation. *J Clin Microbiol* 2002, 40, 2509-2512.

[239] Imperiale, BR; Cataldi, AA; Morcillo, NS. Rapid detection of multidrug-resistant *Mycobacterium tuberculosis* by multiplex allele-specific polymerase chain reaction. *Int J Tuberc Lung Dis* 2011, 15, 496-501.

[240] Vadwai, V; Shetty, A; Rodrigues, C. Multiplex allele specific PCR for rapid detection of extensively drug resistant tuberculosis. *Tuberculosis (Edinburgh)* 2012, 92, 236-242.

[241] Ruiz, M; Torres, MJ; Llanos, AC; Arroyo, A; Palomares, JC; Aznar, J. Direct detection of rifampin- and isoniazid-resistant *Mycobacterium tuberculosis* in auramine-rhodamine-positive sputum specimens by real-time PCR. *J Clin Microbiol* 2004, 42, 1585-1589.

[242] Moure, R; Muñoz, L; Torres, M; Santin, M; Martín, R; Alcaide, F. Rapid detection of *Mycobacterium tuberculosis* complex and rifampin

resistance in smear-negative clinical samples by use of an integrated real-time PCR method. *J Clin Microbiol* 2011, 49, 1137-1139.
[243] Halse, TA; Edwards, J; Cunningham, PL; Wolfgang, WJ; Dumas, NB; Escuyer, VE; Musser, KA. Combined real-time PCR and *rpoB* gene pyrosequencing for rapid identification of *Mycobacterium tuberculosis* and determination of rifampin resistance directly in clinical specimens. *J Clin Microbiol* 2010, 48, 1182-1188.
[244] Lee, AS; Ong, DC. Molecular diagnostic methods for the detection of *Mycobacterium tuberculosis* resistance: the potential of high-resolution melting analysis. *Expert Rev Anti Infect Ther* 2012, 10, 1075-1077.
[245] Ramirez, MV; Cowart, KC; Campbell, PJ; Morlock, GP; Sikes, D; Winchell, JM; Posey, JE. Rapid detection of multidrug-resistant *Mycobacterium tuberculosis* by use of real-time PCR and high-resolution melt analysis. *J Clin Microbiol* 2010, 48, 4003-4009.
[246] Lee, AS; Ong, DC; Wong, JC; Siu, GK; Yam, WC. High-resolution melting analysis for the rapid detection of fluoroquinolone and streptomycin resistance in *Mycobacterium tuberculosis*. *PLoS One* 2012, 7, article no. e31934.
[247] Pholwat, S; Heysell, S; Stroup S; Foongladda, S; Houpt, E. Rapid first- and second-line drug susceptibility assay for *Mycobacterium tuberculosis* isolates by use of quantitative PCR. *J Clin Microbiol* 2011, 49, 69-75.
[248] Choi, JH; Lee, KW; Kang, HR; Hwang, YI; Jang, S; Kim, DG; Kim, CH; Hyun, IG; Shin, TR; Park, SM; Lee, MG; Lee, CY; Park, YB; Jung, KS. Clinical efficacy of direct DNA sequencing analysis on sputum specimens for early detection of drug-resistant *Mycobacterium tuberculosis* in a clinical setting. *Chest* 2010, 137, 393-400.
[249] Garcia-Sierra, N; Lacoma, A; Prat, C; Haba, L; Maldonado, J; Ruiz-Manzano, J; Gavin, P; Samper, S; Ausina, V; Dominguez, J. Pyrosequencing for rapid molecular detection of rifampin and isoniazid resistance in *Mycobacterium tuberculosis* strains and clinical specimens. *J Clin Microbiol* 2011, 49, 3683-3686.
[250] Pérez-Osorio, AC; Boyle, DS; Ingham, ZK; Ostash, A; Gautom, RK; Colombel, C; Houze, Y; Leader, BT. Rapid identification of mycobacteria and drug-resistant *Mycobacterium tuberculosis* by use of a single multiplex PCR and DNA sequencing. *J Clin Microbiol* 2012, 50, 326-336.
[251] Engström, A; Morcillo, N; Imperiale, B; Hoffner, SE; Juréen, P. Detection of first- and second-line drug resistance in *Mycobacterium*

tuberculosis clinical isolates by pyrosequencing. *J Clin Microbiol* 2012, 50, 2026-2033.

[252] Saunders, NJ; Trivedi, UH; Thomson, ML; Doig, C; Laurenson, IF; Blaxter, ML. Deep resequencing of serial sputum isolates of *Mycobacterium tuberculosis* during therapeutic failure due to poor compliance reveals stepwise mutation of key resistance genes on an otherwise stable genetic background. *J Infect* 2011, 62, 212-217.

[253] Sun, G; Luo, T; Yang, C; Dong, X; Li, J; Zhu, Y; Zheng, H; Tian, W; Wang, S; Barry, CE 3rd; Mei, J; Gao, Q. Dynamic population changes in *Mycobacterium tuberculosis* during acquisition and fixation of drug resistance in patients. *J Infect Dis* 2012, 206, 1724-1733.

[254] Ling, DI; Zwerling, AA; Pai, M. GenoType MTBDR assays for the diagnosis of multidrug-resistant tuberculosis: a meta-analysis. *Eur Respir J* 2008, 32, 1165-1174.

[255] Hauck, Y; Fabre, M; Vergnaud, G; Soler, C; Pourcel, C. Comparison of two commercial assays for the characterization of *rpoB* mutations in *Mycobacterium tuberculosis* and description of new mutations conferring weak resistance to rifampicin. *J Antimicrob Chemother* 2009, 64, 259-262.

[256] Al-Mutairi, N; Ahmad, S; Mokaddas, E. Performance comparison of four methods for rapid detection of multidrug-resistant *Mycobacterium tuberculosis* strains. *Int J Tuberc Lung Dis* 2011, 15, 110-115.

[257] Cooksey, RC; Morlock, GP; Glickman, S; Crawford, JT. Evaluation of a line probe assay kit for characterization of *rpoB* mutations in rifampin-resistant *Mycobacterium tuberculosis* isolates from New York City. *J Clin Microbiol* 1997, 35, 1281-1283.

[258] Hillemann, D; Rusch-Gerdes, S; Richter, E. Evaluation of the Genotype MTBDR*plus* assay for rifampin and isoniazid susceptibility testing of *Mycobacterium tuberculosis* strains and clinical specimens. *J Clin Microbiol* 2007, 45, 2635-2640.

[259] Mitarai, S; Kato, S; Ogata, H; Aono, A; Chikamatsu, K; Mizuno, K; Toyota, E; Sejimo, A; Suzuki, K; Yoshida, S; Saito, T; Moriya, A; Fujita, A; Sato, S; Matsumoto, T; Ano, H; Suetake, T; Kondo, Y; Kirikae, T; Mori, T. Comprehensive multicenter evaluation of a new line probe assay kit for identification of *Mycobacterium* species and detection of drug-resistant *Mycobacterium tuberculosis*. *J Clin Microbiol* 2012, 50, 884-890.

[260] Bang, H; Park, S; Hwang, J; Jin, H; Cho, E; Kim, DY; Song, T; Shamputa, IC; Via, LE; Barry, CE 3rd; Cho, SN; Lee, H. Improved

rapid molecular diagnosis of multidrug-resistant tuberculosis using a new reverse hybridization assay, REBA MTB-MDR. *J Med Microbiol* 2011, 60, 1447-1454.

[261] Sekiguchi, JI; Nakamura, T; Miyoshi-Akiyama, T; Kirikae, F; Kobayashi, I; Augustynowicz-Kopec, E; Zwolska, Z; Morita, K; Suetake, T; Yoshida, H; Kato, S; Mori, T; Kirikae, T. Development and evaluation of a line probe assay for rapid identification of *pncA* mutations in pyrazinamide-resistant *Mycobacterium tuberculosis* strains. *J Clin Microbiol* 2007, 45, 2802-2807.

[262] Giannoni, F; Iona, E; Sementilli, F; Brunori, L; Pardini, M; Migliori, GB; Orefici, G; Fattorini, L. Evaluation of a new line probe assay for rapid identification of *gyrA* mutations in *Mycobacterium tuberculosis*. *J Clin Microbiol* 2005, 49, 2928-2933.

[263] Ando, H; Mitarai, S; Kondo, Y; Suetake, T; Kato, S; Mori, T; Kirikae, T. Evaluation of a line probe assay for the rapid detection of *gyrA* mutations associated with fluoroquinolone resistance in multidrug-resistant *Mycobacterium tuberculosis*. *J Med Microbiol* 2011, 60, 184-188.

[264] Hillemann, D; Rusch-Gerdes, S; Richter, E. Feasibility of the GenoType MTBDR*sl* assay for fluoroquinolone, amikacin-capreomycin and ethambutol resistance testing of *Mycobacterium tuberculosis* strains and clinical specimens. *J Clin Microbiol* 2009, 47, 1767-1772.

[265] World health Organization. Molecular line probe assays for the rapid screening of patients at risk of multidrug-resistant tuberculosis (MDR-TB). Policy statement. WHO, Geneva, Switzerland. http//whqlibdoc.who.int/tb/laboratory/pa_policy.pdf. 2008, WHO, 2008.

[266] Morgan, M; Kalantri, S; Flores, L; Pai, M. A commercial line probe assay for the rapid detection of rifampicin resistance in *Mycobacterium tuberculosis*: a systematic review and meta-analysis. *BMC Infect Dis* 2005, 5, article no. 62.

[267] Seoudi, N; Mitchell, SL; Brown, TJ; Dashti, F; Amin, AK; Drobniewski, FA. Rapid molecular detection of tuberculosis and rifampicin drug resistance: retrospective analysis of a national U.K. molecular service over the last decade. *Thorax* 2012, 67, 361-367.

[268] Albert, H; Bwanga, F; Mukkada, S; Nyesiga, B; Ademun, JP; Lukyamuzi, G; Haile, M; Hoffner, S; Joloba, M; O'Brien, R. Rapid screening of MDR-TB using molecular line probe assay is feasible in Uganda. *BMC Infect Dis* 2010, 10, article no. 41.

[269] Skenders, GK; Holtz, TH; Riekstina, V; Leimane, V. Implementation of the INNO-LiPA Rif. TB® line-probe assay in rapid detection of multidrug-resistant tuberculosis in Latvia. *Int J Tuberc Lung Dis* 2011, 15, 1546-1552.

[270] Barnard, M; Albert, H; Coetzee, G; O'Brien, R; Bosman, ME. Rapid molecular screening for multidrug-resistant tuberculosis in a high-volume public health laboratory in South Africa. *Am J Respir Crit Care Med* 2008, 177, 787-792.

[271] Dorman, SE; Chihota, VN; Lewis, JJ; van der Meulen, M; Mathema, B; Beylis, N; Fielding, KL; Grant, AD; Churchyard, GJ. Genotype MTBDR*plus* for direct detection of *Mycobacterium tuberculosis* and drug resistance in strains from gold miners in South Africa. *J Clin Microbiol* 2012, 50, 1189-1194.

[272] Mironova, S; Pimkina, E; Kontsevaya, I; Nikolayevskyy, V; Balabanova, Y; Skenders, G; Kummik, T; Drobniewski, F. Performance of the GenoType® MTBDRPlus assay in routine settings: a multicenter study. *Eur J Clin Microbiol Infect Dis* 2012, 31, 1381-1387.

[273] Crudu, V; Stratan, E; Romancenco, E; Allerheiligen, V; Hillemann, A; Moraru, N. First evaluation of an improved assay for molecular genetic detection of tuberculosis as well as rifampin and isoniazid resistances. *J Clin Microbiol* 2012, 50, 1264-1269.

[274] Barnard, M; Gey van Pittius, NC; van Helden, PD; Bosman, M; Coetzee, G; Warren, RM. The diagnostic performance of the GenoType MTBDR*plus* version 2 line probe assay is equivalent to that of the Xpert MTB/RIF assay. *J Clin Microbiol* 2012, 50, 3712-3716.

[275] Via, LE; Cho, SN; Hwang, S; Bang, H; Park, SK; Kang, HS; Jeon, D; Min, SY; Oh, T; Kim, Y; Kim, YM; Rajan, V; Wong, SY; Shamputa, IC; Carroll, M; Goldfeder, L; Lee, SA; Holland, SM; Eum, S; Lee, H; Barry, CE 3rd. Polymorphisms associated with resistance and cross-resistance to aminoglycosides and capreomycin in *Mycobacterium tuberculosis* isolates from South Korean Patients with drug-resistant tuberculosis. *J Clin Microbiol* 2010, 48, 402-411.

[276] Said, HM; Kock, MM; Ismail, NA; Baba, K; Omar, SV; Osman, AG; Hoosen, AA; Ehlers, MM. Evaluation of the GenoType MTBDR*sl* assay for susceptibility testing of second-line anti-tuberculosis drugs. *Int J Tuberc Lung Dis* 2012, 16, 104-109.

[277] Lacoma, A; García-Sierra, N; Prat, C; Maldonado, J; Ruiz-Manzano, J; Haba, L; Gavin, P; Samper, S; Ausina, V; Domínguez, J. GenoType MTBDR*sl* for molecular detection of second-line-drug and ethambutol

resistance in *Mycobacterium tuberculosis* strains and clinical samples. *J Clin Microbiol* 2012, 50, 30-36.

[278] Miotto, P; Cabibbe, AM; Mantegani, P; Borroni, E; Fattorini, L; Tortoli, E; Migliori, GB; Cirillo, DM. GenoType MTBDR*sl* performance on clinical samples with diverse genetic background. *Eur Respir J* 2012, 40, 690-698.

[279] Ignatyeva, O; Kontsevaya, I; Kovalyov, A; Balabanova, Y; Nikolayevskyy, V; Toit, K; Dragan, A; Maxim, D; Mironova, S; Kummik, T; Muntean, I; Koshkarova, E; Drobniewski, F. Detection of resistance to second-line antituberculosis drugs by use of the genotype MTBDR*sl* assay: a multicenter evaluation and feasibility study. *J Clin Microbiol* 2012, 50, 1593-1597.

[280] Barnard, M; Warren, R; Van Pittius, NG; van Helden, P; Bosman, M; Streicher, E; Coetzee, G; O'Brien, R. GenoType MTBDR*sl* Line Probe assay shortens time to diagnosis of XDR-TB in a high-throughput diagnostic laboratory. *Am J Respir Crit Care Med* 2012, 186, 1298-1305.

[281] Visser, ME; Stead, MC; Walzl, G; Warren, R; Schomaker, M; Grewal, HM; Swart, EC; Maartens, G. Baseline predictors of sputum culture conversion in pulmonary tuberculosis: importance of cavities, smoking, time to detection and W-Beijing genotype. *PLoS One* 2012, 7, article no. e29588.

[282] Espinal, MA; Kim, SJ; Suarez, PG; Kam, KM; Khomenko, AG; Migliori, GB; Baez, J; Kochi, A; Dye, C; Raviglione M. Standard short-course chemotherapy for drug-resistant tuberculosis: treatment outcomes in 6 countries. *JAMA* 2000, 283, 2537-2545.

[283] Escalante, P; Graviss, EA; Griffith, DE; Musser, JM; Awe, RJ. Treatment of isoniazid-resistant tuberculosis in southeastern Texas. *Chest* 2001, 119, 1730-1736.

[284] Jacobson, KR; Theron, D; Victor, TC; Streicher, EM; Warren, RM; Murray, MB. Treatment outcomes of isoniazid-resistant tuberculosis patients, Western Cape Province, South Africa. *Clin Infect Dis* 2011, 53, 369-372.

[285] Gegia, M; Cohen, T; Kalandadze, I; Vashakidze, L; Furin, J. Outcomes among tuberculosis patients with isoniazid resistance in Georgia, 2007-2009. *Int J Tuberc Lung Dis* 2012, 16, 812-816.

[286] Menzies, D; Benedetti, A; Paydar, A; Royce, S; Madhukar, P; Burman, W; Vernon, A; Lienhardt, C. Standardized treatment of active tuberculosis in patients with previous treatment and/or with mono-

resistant to isoniazid: a systematic review and meta-analysis. *PLoS Med* 2009, 6, article no. e1000150.

[287] Lew, W; Pai, M; Oxlade, O; Martin, D; Menzies, D. Initial drug resistance and tuberculosis treatment outcomes: systematic review and meta-analysis. *Ann Intern Med* 2008, 149, 123-134.

[288] L. Heifets, L. Susceptibility testing of *Mycobacterium tuberculosis* to pyrazinamide. *J Med Microbiol* 2002, 51, 11-12.

[289] Yee, DP; Menzies, D; Brassard, P. Clinical outcomes of pyrazinamide-monoresistant *Mycobacterium tuberculosis* in Quebec. *Int J Tuberc Lung Dis* 2012, 16, 604-609.

[290] Kurbatova, EV; Cavanaugh, JS; Shah, NS; Wright, A; Kim, H; Metchock, B; Van Deun, A; Barrera, L; Boulahbal, F; Richter, E; Martín-Casabona, N; Arias, F; Zemanova, I; Drobniewski, F; Santos Silva, A; Coulter, C; Lumb, R; Cegielski, JP. Rifampicin-resistant *Mycobacterium tuberculosis*: susceptibility to isoniazid and other anti-tuberculosis drugs. *Int J Tuberc Lung Dis* 2012,16, 355-357.

[291] World Helath Organization, "Guidelines for the programmatic management of drug-resistant tuberculosis. Emergency update 2008," *WHO/HTM/TB/2008.402.* Geneva, Switzerland. WHO, 2008.

[292] Park, MM; Davis, AL; Schluger, NW; Cohen, H; Rom, WN. Outcome of MDR-TB patients, 1983-1993: prolonged survival with appropriate therapy. *Am J Respir Crit Care Med* 1996, 153, 317-324.

[293] Johnston, JC; Shahidi, NC; Sadatsafavi, M; Fitzgerald, JM. Treatment outcomes of multidrug-resistant tuberculosis: a systematic review and meta-analysis. *PLoS One* 2009, 4, article no. e6914.

[294] Caminero, JA; Sotgiu, G; Zumla, A; Migliori, GB. Best drug treatment for multidrug-resistant and extensively drug-resistant tuberculosis. *Lancet Infect Dis* 2010, 10, 621-629.

[295] Field, SK; Fisher, D; Jarand, JM; Cowie, RL. New treatment options for multidrug-resistant tuberculosis. *Ther Adv Respir Dis* 2012, 6, 255-268.

[296] Suarez, PG; Floyd, K; Portocarrero, J; Alarcón, E; Rapiti, E; Ramos, G; Bonilla, C; Sabogal, I; Aranda, I; Dye, C; Raviglione, M; Espinal, MA. Feaibility and cost-effectiveness of standardized second-line drug treatment for chronic tuberculosis patients: a national cohort study in Peru. *Lancet* 2002, 359, 1980-1989.

[297] Caminero, JA. Treatment of multidrug-resistant tuberculosis: evidence and controversies. *Int J Tuberc Lung Dis* 2006, 10, 829-837.

[298] Falzon, D; Jaramillo, E; Schünemann, HJ; Arentz, M; Bauer, M; Bayona, J; Blanc, L; Caminero, JA; Daley, CL; Duncombe, C; Fitzpatrick, C; Gebhard, A; Getahun, H; Henkens, M; Holtz, TH; Keravec, J; Keshavjee, S; Khan, AJ; Kulier, R; Leimane, V; Lienhardt, C; Lu, C; Mariandyshev, A; Migliori, GB; Mirzayev, F; Mitnick, CD; Nunn, P; Nwagboniwe, G; Oxlade, O; Palmero, D; Pavlinac, P; Quelapio, MI; Raviglione, MC; Rich, ML; Royce, S; Rüsch-Gerdes, S; Salakaia, A; Sarin, R; Sculier, D; Varaine, F; Vitoria, M; Walson, JL; Wares, F; Weyer, K; White, RA; Zignol, M. WHO guidelines for the programmatic management of drug-resistant tuberculosis: 2011 update. *Eur Resp J* 2011, 38, 516-528.

[299] Van Deun, A; Maug, AK; Salim, MA; Das, PK; Sarker, MR; Daru, P; Rieder, HL. Short, highly effective and inexpensive standardised treatment of multidrug-resistant tuberculosis. *Am J Respir Crit Care Med* 2010, 182, 684-692.

[300] Sotgiu, G; Centis, R; D'Ambrosio, L; Alffenaar, J; Anger, H; Caminero, J; Castiglia, P; De Lorenzo, S; Ferrara, G; Koh, W; Schecter, G; Shim, T; Singla, R; Skrahina, A; Spanevello, A; Udwadia, Z; Villar, M; Zampogna, E; Zellweger, J; Zumla, A; Migliori, GB. Efficacy, safety and tolerability of linezolid containing regimens in treating MDR-TB and XDR-TB: systematic review and meta-analysis. *Eur Respir J* 2012, 40, 1430-1442.

[301] Katiyar, SK; Bihari, S; Prakash, S; Mamtani, M; Kulkarni, H. A randomized controlled trial of high-dose isoniazid adjuvant therapy for multidrug-resistant tuberculosis. *Int J Tuberc Lung Dis* 2008, 12, 129-145.

[302] Shin, SS; Pasechnikov, AD; Gelmanova, IY; Peremitin, GG; Strelis, AK; Mishustin, S; Barnashov, A; Karpeichik, Y; Andreev, YG; Golubchikova, VT; Tonkel, TP; Yanova, GV; Yedilbayev, A; Rich, ML; Mukherjee, JS; Furin, JJ; Atwood, S; Farmer, PE; Keshavjee, S. Adverse reactions among patients being treated for MDR-TB in Tomsk, Russia. *Int J Tuberc Lung Dis* 2007, 11, 1314-1320.

[303] Sturdy, A; Goodman, A; José, RJ; Loyse, A; O'Donoghue, M; Kon, OM; Dedicoat, MJ; Harrison, TS; John, L; Lipman, M; Cooke, GS. Multidrug-resistant tuberculosis (MDR-TB) treatment in the UK: a study of injectable use and toxicity in practice. *J Antimicrob Chemother* 2011, 66, 1815-1820.

[304] Holtz, TH; Sternberg, M; Kammerer, S; Laserson, KF; Riekstina, V; Zarovska, E; Skripconoka, V; Wells, CD; Leimane, V. Time to sputum

culture conversion in multidrug-resistant tuberculosis: predictors and relationship to treatment outcome. *Ann Intern Med* 2006, 144, 650-659.

[305] Chiang, CY; Caminero, J; Enarson, DA. Reporting on multidrug-resistant tuberculosis: a proposed definition for the treatment outcome 'failed'. *Int J Tuberc Lung Dis* 2009, 13, 548-550.

[306] Gammino, VM; Taylor, AB; Rich, ML; Bayona, J; Becerra, MC; Bonilla, C; Gelmanova, I; Hollo, V; Jaramillo, E; Keshavjee, S; Leimane, V; Mitnick, CD; Quelapio, MI; Riektsina, V; Tupasi, TE; Wells, CD; Zignol, M; Cegielski, PJ. Bacteriologic monitoring of multidrug-resistant tuberculosis patients in five DOTS-Plus pilot projects. *Int J Tuberc Lung Dis* 2011, 15, 1315-1322.

[307] Kang, MW; Kim, HK; Choi, YS; Kim, K; Shim, YM; Koh, WJ; Kim, J. Surgical treatment for multidrug-resistant and extensive drug-resistant tuberculosis. *Ann Thorac Surg* 2010, 89, 1597-1602.

[308] Kempker, RR; Vashakidze, S; Solomonia, N; Dzidzikashvili, N; Blumberg, HM. Surgical treatment of drug-resistant tuberculosis. *Lancet Infect Dis* 2012, 12, 157-166.

[309] Gegia, M; Kalandadze, I; Kempker, RR; Magee, MJ; Blumberg, HM. Adjunctive surgery improves treatment outcomes among patients with multidrug-resistant and extensively drug-resistant tuberculosis. *Int J Infect Dis* 2012, 16, e391-e396.

[310] Ahuja, SD; Ashkin, D; Avendano, M; Banerjee, R; Bauer, M; Bayona, JN; Becerra, MC; Benedetti, A; Burgos, M; Centis, R; Chan, ED; Chiang, CY; Cox, H; D'Ambrosio, L; DeRiemer, K; Dung, NH; Enarson, D; Falzon, D; Flanagan, K; Flood, J; Garcia-Garcia, ML; Gandhi, N; Granich, RM; Hollm-Delgado, MG; Holtz, TH; Iseman, MD; Jarlsberg, LG; Keshavjee, S; Kim, HR; Koh, WJ; Lancaster, J; Lange, C; de Lange, WC; Leimane, V; Leung, CC; Li, J; Menzies, D; Migliori, GB; Mishustin, SP; Mitnick, CD; Narita, M; O'Riordan, P; Pai, M; Palmero, D; Park, SK; Pasvol, G; Peña, J; Pérez-Guzmán, C; Quelapio, MI; Ponce-de-Leon, A; Riekstina, V; Robert, J; Royce, S; Schaaf, HS; Seung, KJ; Shah, L; Shim, TS; Shin, SS; Shiraishi, Y; Sifuentes-Osornio, J; Sotgiu, G; Strand, MJ; Tabarsi, P; Tupasi, TE; van Altena, R; Van der Walt, M; Van der Werf, TS; Vargas, MH; Viiklepp, P; Westenhouse, J; Yew, WW; Yim, JJ; Collaborative Group for Meta-Analysis of Individual Patient Data in MDR-TB. Multidrug resistant pulmonary tuberculosis treatment regimens and patient outcomes: an individual patient data meta-analysis of 9,153 patients. *PLoS Med* 2012, 9, article no. e1001300.

[311] World Health Organization, "Guidelines for the programmatic management of drug-resistant tuberculosis. 2011 update," Geneva, Switzerland, http://whqlibdoc.who.int/publications/2011/9789241501583_eng.pdf. WHO, 2011.

[312] Sotgiu, G; Ferrara, G; Matteelli, A; Richardson, MD; Centis, R; Ruesch-Gerdes, S; Toungoussova, O; Zellweger, JP; Spanevello, A; Cirillo, D; Lange, C; Migliori, GB. Epidemiology and clinical management of XDR-TB: a systematic review by TBNET. *Eur Respir J* 2009, 33, 871-881.

[313] Centers for Disease Control and Prevention (CDC). Plan to combat extensively drug-resistant tuberculosis: recommendations of the Federal Tuberculosis Task Force. *Mor Mort Weekly Rep* 2009, 58(RR03), 1-43.

[314] Migliori, GB; Sotgiu, G; Lange, C; Centis, R. Extensively drug-resistant tuberculosis: back to the future. *Eur Respir J* 2010, 36, 475-477.

[315] Amaral, L; Viveiros, M. Why thioridazine in combination with antibiotics cures extensively drug-resistant *Mycobacterium tuberculosis* infections. *Int J Antimicrob Agents* 2012, 39, 376-380.

[316] Flipo, M; Desroses, M; Lecat-Guillet, N; Dirié, B; Carette, X; Leroux, F; Piveteau, C; Demirkaya, F; Lens, Z; Rucktooa, P; Villeret, V; Christophe, T; Jeon, HK; Locht, C; Brodin, P; Déprez, B; Baulard, AR; Willand, N. Ethionamide boosters: synthesis, biological activity, and structure-activity relationships of a series of 1,2,4-oxadiazole EthR inhibitors. *J Med Chem* 2011, 54, 2994-3010.

[317] Migliori, GB; Besozzi, G; Girardi, E; Kliiman, K; Lange, C; Toungoussova, OS; Ferrara, G; Cirillo, DM; Gori, A; Matteelli, A; Spanevello, A; Codecasa, LR; Raviglione, MC; SMIRA/TBNET Study Group. Clinical and operational value of the extensively drug-resistant tuberculosis definition. *Eur Respir J* 2007, 30, 623-626.

[318] Marquez, L; Starke, JR. Diagnosis and management of TB in children: an update. *Expert Rev Anti Infect Ther* 2011, 9, 1157-1168.

[319] Perez-Velez, CM. Pediatric tuberculosis: new guidelines and recommendations. *Curr Opin Pediatr* 2012, 24, 319-328.

[320] Seddon, JA; Hesseling, AC; Marias, BJ; McIlleron, H; Peloquin, CA; Donald, PR; Schaaf, SH. Pediatric use of second-line anti-tuberculosis agents: a review. *Tuberculosis (Edinburgh)* 2012, 92, 9-17.

[321] Hesseling, AC; Kim, S; Madhi, S; Nachman, S; Schaaf, HS; Violari, A; Victor, TC; McSherry, G; Mitchell, C; Cotton, MF; IMPAACT P1041

Team. High prevalence of drug resistance amongst HIV-exposed and -infected children in a tuberculosis prevention trial. *Int J Tuberc Lung Dis* 2012, 16, 192-195.

[322] Seddon, JA; Visser, DH; Bartens, M; Jordaan, AM; Victor, TC; van Furth, AM; Schoeman, JF; Schaaf, HS. Impact of drug resistance on clinical outcome in children with tuberculous meningitis. *Pediatr Infect Dis J* 2012, 31, 711-716.

[323] Meintjes, G; Lawn, SD; Scano, F; Maartens, G; French, MA; Worodria, W; Elliott, JH; Murdoch, D; Wilkinson, RJ; Seyler, C; John, L; Schim van der Loeff, M; Reiss, P; Lyne, L; Janoff, EN; Gilks, C; Colebunders, R; for the International Network for the Study of HIV-associated IRIS. Tuberculosis-associated immune reconstitution inflammatory syndrome: case definitions for use in resource-limited settings. *Lancet Infect Dis* 2008, 8, 516-523.

[324] Scano, F; Vitoria, M; Burman, W; Harries, AD; Gilks, CF; Havlir, D. Management of HIV-infected patients with MDR-TB and XDR-TB in resource-limited settings. *Int J Tuberc Lung Dis* 2008, 12, 1370-1375.

[325] Gandhi, NR; Moll, A; Sturm, AW; Pawinski, R; Govender, T; Lalloo, U; Zeller, K; Andrews, J; Friedland, G. Extensively drug-resistant tuberculosis as a cause of death in patients co-infected with tuberculosis and HIV in a rural area of South Africa. *Lancet* 2006, 368, 1575-1580.

[326] Seung, KJ; Omatayo, DB; Keshavjee, S; Furin, JJ; Farmer, PE; Satti, H. Early outcomes of MDR-TB treatment in a high prevalence setting in Southern Africa. *PLoS One* 2009, 4, article no. e7186.

[327] Satti, H; McLaughlin, MM; Hedt-Gauthier, B; Atwood, SS; Omotayo, DB; Ntlamelle, L; Seung, KJ. Outcomes of multidrug-resistant tuberculosis treatment with early initiation of antiretroviral therapy for HIV co-infected patients in Lesotho. *PLoS One* 2012, 7, article no. e46943.

[328] Gandhi, NR; Shah, NS; Andrews, JR; Vella, V; Moll, AP; Scott, M; Weissman, D; Marra, C; Lalloo, UG; Friedland, GH; Tugela Ferry Care and Research (TF CARES) Collaboration. HIV-coinfection in multidrug- and extensively drug-resistant tuberculosis results in high early mortality. *Am J Respir Care Crit Med* 2010, 181, 80-86.

[329] Palomino, JC; Martin, A. Is repositioning of drugs a viable alternative in the treatment of tuberculosis? *J Antimicrob Chemother* 2013, 68, 275-283.

[330] Koul, A; Arnoult, E; Lounis, N; Guillemont, J; Andries, K. The challenge of new drug discovery for tuberculosis. *Nature* 2011, 469, 483-490.

[331] Ma, Z; Lienhardt, C; McIlleron, H; Nunn, AJ; Wang, X. Global tuberculosis drug development pipeline: the need and the reality. *Lancet* 2010, 375, 2100-2109.

[332] Ginsberg, AM. Drugs in development for tuberculosis. *Drugs* 2010, 70, 2201-2214.

[333] Cole, ST; Riccardi, G. New tuberculosis drugs on the horizon. *Curr Opin Microbiol* 2011, 14, 570-576.

[334] Grosset, JH; Singer, TG; Bishai, WR. New drugs for the treatment of tuberculosis: hope and reality. *Int J Tuberc Lung Dis* 2012, 16, 1005-1014.

[335] Van Deun, A; Salim, MA; Das, AP; Bastian, I; Portaels, F. Results of a standardized regimen for multidrug-resistant tuberculosis in Bangladesh. *Int J Tuberc Lung Dis* 2004, 8, 560-567.

[336] Schaaf, HS; Moll, AP; Dheda, K. Multidrug- and extensively drug-resistant tuberculosis in Africa and South America: epidemiology, diagnosis and management in adults and children. *Clin Chest Med* 2009, 30, 667-683.

[337] Mitchison, D; Fourie, P. The near future: improving the activity of rifamycins and pyrazinamide. *Tuberculosis (Edinburgh)* 2010, 90, 177-181.

[338] Wilkins, JJ; Savic, RM; Karlsson, MO; Langdon, G; McIlleron, H; Pillai, G; Smith, PJ; Simonsson, US. Population pharmacokinetics of rifampin in pulmonary tuberculosis patients, including a semimechanistic model to describe variable absorption. *Antimicrob Agents Chemother* 2008, 52, 2138-2148.

[339] Diacon, AH; Partientia, RF; Venter, A; van Helden, PD; Smith, PJ; McIlleron, H; Maritz, JS; Donald, PR. Early bactericidal activity of high-dose rifampin in patients with pulmonary tuberculosis evidenced by positive sputum smears. *Antimicrob Agents Chemother* 2007, 51, 2994-2996.

[340] Steingart, KR; Jotblad, S; Robsky, K; Deck, D; Hopewell, PC; Huang, D; Nahid, P. Higher-dose rifampin for the treatment of pulmonary tuberculosis: a systematic review. *Int J Tuberc Lung Dis* 2011, 15, 305-316.

[341] Dorman, SE; Goldberg, S; Stout, JE; Muzanyi, G; Johnson, JL; Weiner, M; Bozeman, L; Heilig, CM; Feng, PJ; Moro, R; Narita, M; Nahid, P;

Ray, S; Bates, E; Haile, B; Nuermberger, EL; Vernon, A; Schluger, NW; Tuberculosis Trials Consortium. Substitution of rifapentine for rifampin during intensive phase treatment of pulmonary tuberculosis: study 29 of the tuberculosis trials consortium. *J Infect Dis* 2012, 206, 1030-1040.

[342] Sirgel, FA; Fourie, PB; Donald, PR; Padayatchi, N; Rustomjee, R; Levin, J; Roscigno, G; Norman, J; McIlleron, H; Mitchison, DA. The early bactericidal activities of rifampin and rifapentine in pulmonary tuberculosis. *Am J Respir Crit Care Med* 2005, 172, 128-135.

[343] Rosenthal, IM; Zhang, M; Almeida, D; Grosset, JH; Nuermberger, EL. Isoniazid or moxifloxacin in rifapentine-based regimens for experimental tuberculosis. *Am J Respir Crit Care Med* 2008, 178, 989-993

[344] ClinicalTrials.gov, "A controlled trial of a 4-month quinolone-containing regimen for the treatment of pulmonary tuberculosis," *Trial Identifier*: NCT00216385.

[345] ClinicalTrials.gov, "Controlled comparison of two moxifloxacin-containing treatment shortening regimens in pulmonary tuberculosis," *Trial Identifier*: NCT00864383.

[346] Balasubramanian, V; Solapure, S; Gaonkar, S; Mahesh Kumar, KN; Shandil, RK; Deshpande, A; Kumar, N; Vishwas, KG; Panduga, V; Reddy, J; Ganguly, S; Louie, A; Drusano, GL. Effect of coadministration of moxifloxacin and rifampin on *Mycobacterium tuberculosis* in a murine aerosol infection model. *Antimicrob Agents Chemother* 2012, 56, 3054-3057.

[347] Devasia, RA; Blackman, A; Gebretsadik, T; Griffin, M; Shintani, A; May, C; Smith, T; Hooper, N; Maruri, F; Warkentin, J; Mitchel, E; Sterling, TR. Fluoroquinolone resistance in *Mycobacterium tuberculosis*: the effect of duration and timing of fluoroquinolone exposure. *Am J Respir Crit Care Med* 2009, 180, 365-370.

[348] Chen, TC; Lu, PL; Lin, CY; Lin, WR; Chen, YH. Fluoroquinolones are associated with delayed treatment and resistance in tuberculosis: a systematic review and meta-analysis. *Int J Infect Dis* 2011, 15, e211-e216.

[349] Shen, GH; Tsao, TC; Kao, SJ; Lee, JJ; Chen, YH; Hsieh, WC; Hsu, GJ; Hsu, YT; Huang, CT; Lau, YJ; Tsao, SM; Hsueh, PR. Does empirical treatment of community-acquired pneumonia with fluoroquinolones delay tuberculosis treatment and result in fluoroquinolone resistance in

Mycobacterium tuberculosis? Controversies and solutions. *Int J Antimicrob Agents* 2012, 39, 201-205.

[350] Migliori, GB; Langendam, MW; D'Ambrosio, L; Centis, R; Blasi, F; Huitric, E; Manissero, D; van der Werf, MJ. Protecting the tuberculosis drug pipeline: stating the case for the rational use of fluoroquinolones. *Eur Respir J* 2012, 40, 814-822.

[351] Hugonnet, J-E; Tremblay, LW; Boshoff, HI; Barry, CE 3rd; Blanchard, JS. Meropenem-clavulanate is effective against extensively drug-resistant *Mycobacterium tuberculosis*. *Science* 2009, 323, 1215-1218.

[352] Veziris, C; Truffat, J-L; Mainardi, Jarlier, V. Activity of carbapenems combined with clavulanate agasinst murine tuberculosis. *Antimicrob Agents Chemother* 2011, 55, 2597-2600.

[353] Barry, VC; Belton, JG; Conalty ML; Denneny, JM; Edward, DW; O'Sullivan, JF; Towmey, D; Winder, F. A new series of phenazines (rimino-compounds) with high anti-tuberculosis activity. *Nature* 1957, 179, 1013-1015.

[354] Williams, K; Minkowski, A; Amoabeng, O; Peloquin, CA; Taylor, D; Andries, K; Wallis, RS; Mdluli, KE; Nuermberger, EL. Sterilizing activities of novel combinations lacking first- and second-line drugs in a murine model of tuberculosis. *Antimicrob Agents Chemother* 2012, 56, 3114-3120.

[355] Cholo, MC; Steel, HC; Fourie, PB; Germishuizen, WA; Anderson, R. Clofazimine: current status and future prospects. *J Antimicrob Chemother* 2012, 67, 290-298.

[356] Lu, Y; Zheng, M; Wang, B; Fu, L; Zhao, W; Li, P; Xu, J; Zhu, H; Jin, H; Yin, D; Huang, H; Upton, AM; Ma, Z. Clofazimine analogs with efficacy against experimental tuberculosis and reduced potential for accumulation. *Antimicrob Agents Chemother* 2011, 55, 5185-5193.

[357] Dietze, R; Hadad, DJ; McGee, B; Molino, LP; Macielm EL; Peloquinm CA; Johnson, DF; Debanne, SM; Eisenach, K; Boom, WH; Palaci, M; Johnson, JL. Early and extended early bactericidal activity of linezolid in pulmonary tuberculosis. *Am J Respir Crit Care Med* 2008, 178, 1180-1185.

[358] Migliori, GB; Eker, B; Richardson, MD; Sotgiu, G; Zellweger, JP; Skrahina, A; Ortmann, J; Girardi, E; Hoffmann, H; Besozzi, G; Bevilacqua, N; Kirsten, D; Centis, R; Lange, C; TBNET Study Group. A retrospective TBNET assessment of linezolid safety, tolerability and efficacy in multidrug-resistant tuberculosis. *Eur Respir J* 2009, 34, 387-393.

[359] Yew, WW; Chang, KC; Chau, CH. What is the optimal dosage of linezolid in treatment of complicated multidrug-resistant tuberculosis? *Eur Respir* J 2009, 34, 1492-1494.

[360] Villar, M; Sotgiu, G; D'Ambrosio, L; Raymundo, E; Fernandes, L; Barbedo, J; Diogo, N; Lange, C; Centis, R; Migliori, GB. Linezolid safety, tolerability and efficacy to treat multidrug- and extensively drug-resistant tuberculosis. *Eur Respir J* 2011, 38, 730-733.

[361] Nam, HS; Koh, WJ; Kwon, OJ; Cho, SN; Shim, TS. Daily half dose linezolid for intractable multidrug-resistant tuberculosis. *Int J Antimicrob Agents* 2009, 33, 92-93.

[362] Koh, WJ; Kwon, OJ; Gwak, H; Chung, JW; Cho, SN; Kim, WS; Shim, TS. Daily 300 mg dose of linezolid for the treatment of intractable multidrug-resistant and extensively drug-resistant tuberculosis. *J Antimicrob Chemother* 2009, 64, 388-391.

[363] Engohang-Ndong, J; Baillat, D; Aumercier M; Bellefontaine, F; Besra, GS; Locht, C; Baulard, AR. EthR, a repressor of the TetR/CamR family implicated in ethionamide resistance in mycobacteria, octamerizes cooperatively on its operator. *Mol Microbiol* 2004, 51, 175-188.

[364] Dover, LG; Alahari, A; Gratraud, P; Gomes, JM; Bhowruth, V; Reynolds, RC; Besra, GS; Kremer, L. EthA, a common activator of thiocarbamide-containing drugs acting on different mycobacterial targets. *Antimicrob Agents Chemother* 2007, 51, 1055-1063.

[365] Willand, N; Dirié, B; Carette, X; Bifani, P; Singhal, A; Desroses, M; Leroux, F; Willery, E; Mathys, V; Déprez-Poulain, R; Delcroix, G; Frénois, F; Aumercier, M; Locht, C; Villeret, V; Déprez, B; Baulard, AR. Synthetic EthR inhibitors boost antituberculous activity of ethionamide. *Nat Med* 2009, 15, 537-544.

[366] Flipo, M; Desroses, M; Lecat-Guillet, N; Dirié, B; Carette, X; Leroux, F; Piveteau, C; Demirkaya, F; Lens, Z; Rucktooa, P; Villeret, V; Christophe, T; Jeon, HK; Locht, C; Brodin, P; Déprez, B; Baulard, AR; Willand, N. Ethionamide boosters: synthesis, biological activity, and structure-activity relationships of a series of 1,2,4-oxadiazole EthR inhibitors. *J Med Chem* 2011, 54, 2994-3010.

[367] Grau, T; Selchow, P; Tigges, M; Burri, R; Gitzinger, M; Böttger, EC; Fussenegger, M; Sander, P. Phenylethyl butyrate enhances the potency of second-line drugs against clinical isolates of *Mycobacterium tuberculosis*. *Antimicrob Agents Chemother* 2012, 56, 1142-1145.

[368] Flipo, M; Willand, N; Lecat-Guillet, N; Hounsou, C; Desroses, M; Leroux, F; Lens, Z; Villeret, V; Wohlkönig, A; Wintjens, R;

Christophe, T; Kyoung Jeon, H; Locht, C; Brodin, P; Baulard, AR; Déprez, B. Discovery of novel N-phenylphenoxyacetamide derivatives as EthR inhibitors and ethionamide boosters by combining high-throughput screening and synthesis. *J Med Chem* 2012, 55, 6391-6402.

[369] Sharma S; Singh, A. Phenothiazines as anti-tubercular agents: mechanistic insights and clinical implications. *Expert Opin Investig Drugs* 2011, 20, 1665-1676.

[370] Liu, B; Liu, K; Lu, Y; Zhang, D; Yang, T; Li, X; Ma, C; Zheng, M; Wang, B; Zhang, G; Wang, F; Ma, Z; Li, C; Huang, H; Yin, D. Systematic evaluation of structure-activity relationships of the riminophenazine class and discovery of a C2 pyridylamino series for the treatment of multidrug-resistant tuberculosis. *Molecules* 2012, 17, 4545-4559.

[371] Amaral, L; Viveiros, M. Why thioridazine in combination with antibiotics cures extensively drug-resistant *Mycobacterium tuberculosis* infections. *Int J Antimicrob Agents* 2012, 39, 376-380.

[372] Pepper, DJ; Meintjes, GA; McIlleron, H; Wilkinson, RJ. Combined therapy for tuberculosis and HIV-1: the challenge for drug discovery. *Drug Discovery Today* 2007, 12, 980-989.

[373] Andries, K; Verhasselt, P; Guillemont, J; Göhlmann, HW; Neefs, JM; Winkler, H; Van Gestel, J; Timmerman, P; Zhu, M; Lee, E; Williams, P; de Chaffoy, D; Huitric, E; Hoffner, S; Cambau, E; Truffot-Pernot, C; Lounis, N; Jarlier, V. A diarylquinoline drug active on the ATP synthase of *Mycobacterium tuberculosis*. *Science* 2005, 307, 223-227.

[374] Koul, A; Dendouga, N; Vergauwen, K; Molenberghs, B; Vranckx, L; Willebrords, R; Ristic, Z; Lill, H; Dorange, I; Guillemont, J; Bald, D; Andries, K. Diarylquinoline target subunit c of mycobacterial ATP synthase. *Nat Chem Biol* 2007, 3, 323-324.

[375] Huitric, E; Verhasselt, P; Koul, A; Andries, K; Hoffner, S; Andersson, DI. Rates and mechanisms of resistance development in *Mycobacterium tuberculosis* to a novel diarylquinoline ATP synthase inhibitor. *Antimicrob Agents Chemother* 2010, 54, 1022-1028.

[376] Dhillon, J; Andries, K; Phillips, PPJ; Mitchison, DA. Bactericidal activity of the diarylquinoline TMC207 against *Mycobacterium tuberculosis* outside and within cells. *Tuberculosis (Edinburgh)* 2010, 90, 301-305.

[377] Rustomjee, R; Diacon, AH; Allen, J; Venter, A; Reddy, C; Patientia, RF; Mthiyane, TC; De Marez, T; van Heeswijk, R; Kerstens, R; Koul, A; De Beule, K; Donald, PR; McNeeley, DF. Early bactericidal activity

and pharmacokinetics of the diarylquinoline TMC-207 in treatment of pulmonary tuberculosis. *Antimicrob Agents Chemother* 2008, 52, 2831-2835.

[378] Veziris, N; Ibrahim, M; Lounis, N; Chauffour, A; Truffot-Pernot, C; Andries, K; Jarlier, V. A once-weekly R207910-containing regimen exceeds activity of the standard daily regimen in murine tuberculosis. *Am J Respir Crit Care Med* 2009, 179, 75-79.

[379] Ibrahim, M; Truffot-Pernot, C; Andries, K; Jarlier, V; Veziris, N. Sterilizing activity of R207910 (TMC207)-containing regimens in the murine model of tuberculosis. *Am J Respir Crit Care Med* 2009, 180, 553-557.

[380] Dooley, KE; Park, JG; Swindells, S; Allen, R; Haas, DW; Cramer, Y; Aweeka, F; Wiggins, I; Gupta, A; Lizak, P; Qasba, S; van Heeswijk, R; Flexner, C; ACTG 5267 Study Team. Safety, tolerability, and pharmacokinetic interactions of the antituberculous agent TMC207 (bedaquiline) with efavirenz in healthy volunteers: AIDS Clinical Trials Group Study A5267. *J Acquir Immune Defic Syndr* 2012, 59, 455-462.

[381] Lounis, N; Veziris, N; Chauffour, A; Truffot-Pernot, C; Andries, K; Jarlier, V. Combinations of R207910 with drugs used to treat multidrug-resistant tuberculosis have the potential to shorten treatment duration. *Antimicrob Agents Chemother* 2006, 50, 3543-3547.

[382] Shang, S; Shanley, CA; Caraway, ML; Orme, EA; Henao-Tamayo, M; Hascall-Dove, L; Ackart, D; Lenaerts, AJ; Basaraba, RJ; Orme, IM; Ordway, DJ. Activities of TMC207, rifampin, and pyrazinamide against *Mycobacterium tuberculosis* infection in guinea pigs. *Antimicrob Agents Chemother* 2011, 55, 124-131.

[383] Veziris, N; Ibrahim, M; Lounis, N; Andries, K; Jarlier, V. Sterilizing activity of second-line regimens containing TMC207 in a murine model of tuberculosis. *PLoS One* 2011, 6, article no. e17556.

[384] Diacon, AH; Pym, A; Grobusch, M; Patientia, R; Rustomjee, R; Page-Shipp, L; Pistorius, C; Krause, R; Bogoshi, M; Churchyard, G; Venter, A; Allen, J; Palomino, JC; De Marez, T; van Heeswijk, RP; Lounis, N; Meyvisch, P; Verbeeck, J; Parys, W; de Beule, K; Andries, K; Neeley, DF. The diarylquinoline TMC207 for multidrug-resistant tuberculosis. *N Engl J Med* 2009, 360, 2397-2405.

[385] Diacon, AH; Donald, PR; Pym, A; Grobusch, M; Patientia, RF; Mahanyele, R; Bantubani, N; Narasimooloo, R; De Marez, T; van Heeswijk, R; Lounis, N; Meyvisch, P; Andries, K; McNeeley, DF. Randomized pilot trial of eight weeks of bedaquiline (TMC207)

treatment for multidrug-resistant tuberculosis: long-term outcome, tolerability, and effect on emergence of drug resistance. *Antimicrob Agents Chemother* 2012, 56, 3271-3276.

[386] ClinicalTrials.gov. A phase III placebo-controlled, double-blind, randomized trial to evaluate the efficacy and safety of TMC207 in subjects with sputum smear-positive pulmonary infection with multi-drug resistant *Mycobacterium tuberculosis* (MDR-TB). *Trial identifier*: NCT01600963.

[387] Mukherjee, T; Boshoff, H. Nitroimidazoles for the treatment of TB: past, present and future. *Future Med Chem* 2011, 3, 1427-1454.

[388] Manjunatha, UH; Boshoff, H; Dowd, CS; Zhang, L; Albert, TJ; Norton, JE; Daniels, L; Dick, T; Pang, SS; Barry, CE 3rd. Identification of a nitroimidazo-oxazine-specific protein involved in PA-824 resistance in *Mycobacterium tuberculosis*. *Proc Natl Acad Sci USA* 2006, 103, 431-436.

[389] Bashiri, G; Squire, CJ; Moreland, NJ; Baker, EN. Crystal structures of F420-dependent glucose-6-phosphate dehydrogenase FGD1 involved in the activation of the anti-tuberculosis drug candidate PA-824 reveal the basis of coenzyme and substrate binding. *J Biol Chem* 2008, 283, 17531-17541.

[390] Gurumurthy, M; Mukherjee, T; Dowd, CS; Singh, R; Niyomrattanakit, P; Tay, JA; Nayyar, A; Lee, YS; Cherian, J; Boshoff, HI; Dick, T; Barry, CE 3rd; Manjunatha, UH. Substrate specificity of the deazaflavin-dependent nitroreductase from *Mycobacterium tuberculosis* responsible for the bioreductive activation of bicyclic nitroimidazoles. *FEBS J* 2012, 279, 113-125.

[391] Ginsberg, AM; Laurenzi, MW; Rouse, DJ; Whitney, KD; Spigelman, MK. Safety, tolerability, and pharmacokinetics of PA-824 in healthy subjects. *Antimicrob Agents Chemother* 2009, 53, 3720-3725.

[392] Diacon, AH; Dawson, R; Hanekom, M; Narunsky, K; Maritz, SJ; Venter, A; Donald, PR; van Niekerk, C; Whitney, K; Rouse, DJ; Laurenzi, MW; Ginsberg, AM; Spigelman, MK. Early bactericidal activity and pharmacokinetics of PA-824 in smear-positive tuberculosis patients. *Antimicrob Agents Chemother* 2010, 54, 3402-3407.

[393] Singh, R; Manjunatha, U; Boshoff, HI; Ha, YH; Niyomrattanakit, P; Ledwidge, R; Dowd, CS; Lee, IY; Kim, P; Zhang, L; Kang, S; Keller, TH; Jiricek, J; Barry, CE 3rd. PA-824 kills nonreplicating *Mycobacterium tuberculosis* by intracellular NO release. *Science* 2008, 322, 1392-1395.

[394] Ahmad, Z; Peloquin, CA; Singh, RP; Derendorf, H; Tyagi, S; Ginsberg, A; Grosset, JH; Nuermberger, EL. PA-824 exhibits time-dependent activity in a murine model of tuberculosis. *Antimicrob Agents Chemother* 2011, 55, 239-245.

[395] Tyagi, S; Nuermberger, E; Yoshimatsu, T; Williams, K; Rosenthal, I; Lounis, N; Bishai, W; Grosset, J. Bactericidal activity of the nitroimidazopyran PA-824 in a murine model of tuberculosis. *Antimicrob Agents Chemother* 2005, 49, 2289-2293.

[396] Nuermberger, E; Tyagi, S; Tasneen, R; Williams, KN; Almeida, D; Rosenthal, I; Grosset, JH. Powerful bactericidal and sterilizing activity of a regimen containing PA-824, moxifloxacin and pyrazinamide in a murine model of tuberculosis. *Antimicrob Agents Chemother* 2008, 52, 1522-1524.

[397] Tasneen, R; Tyagi, S; Williams, K; Grosset, J; Nuermberger, E. Enhanced bactericidal activity of rifampin and/or pyrazinamide when combined with PA-824 in a murine model of tuberculosis. *Antimicrob Agents Chemother* 2008, 52, 3664-3668.

[398] Diacon, AH; Dawson, R; von Groote-Bidlingmaier, F; Symons, G; Venter, A; Donald, PR; van Niekerk, C; Everitt, D; Winter, H; Becker, P; Mendel, CM; Spigelman, MK. 14-day bactericidal activity of PA-824, bedaquiline, pyrazinamide, and moxifloxacin combinations: a randomised trial. *Lancet* 2012, 380, 986-993.

[399] Tasneen, R; Li, SY; Peloquin, CA; Taylor, D; Williams, KN; Andries, K; Mdluli, KE; Nuermberger, EL. Sterilizing activity of novel TMC207- and PA-824-containing regimens in a murine model of tuberculosis. *Antimicrob Agents Chemother* 2011,55, 5485-5492

[400] ClinicalTrials.gov. A phase II open-label partially randomized trial to evaluate the efficacy, safety and tolerability of the combination of moxifloxacin plus PA-824 plus pyrazinamide after 8 weeks of treatment in adult patients with newly diagnosed drug-sensitive or multi drug-resistant, smear-positive pulmonary tuberculosis. *Trial Identifier*: NCT01498419

[401] ClinicalTrials.gov. A phase 2 trial to evaluate the early bactericidal activity, safety and tolerability of the following: TMC207 plus PA-824 plus pyrazinamide plus clofazimine, TMC207 plus PA-824 plus pyrazinamide, TMC207 plus PA-824 plus clofazimine alone, TMC207 plus pyrazinamide plus clofazimine, pyrazinamide alone and clofazimine alone in adult patients with smear-positive pulmonary tuberculosis. *Trial Identifier*: NCT01691534.

[402] Matsumoto, M; Hashizume, H; Tomishige, T; Kawasaki, M; Tsubouchi, H; Sasaki, H; Shimokawa, Y; Komatsu, M. OPC-67683, a nitro-dihydro-imidazooxazole derivative with promising action against tuberculosis in vitro and in mice. *PLos Med* 2006, 3, article no. e466.

[403] Diacon, AH ; Dawson, R; Hanekom, M; Narunsky, K; Venter, A; Hittel, N; Geiter, LJ; Wells, CD; Paccaly, AJ; Donald, PR. Early bactericidal activity of delamanid (OPC-67683) in smear-positive pulmonary tuberculosis patients. *Int J Tuberc Lung Dis* 2011, 15, 949-954.

[404] Gler, MT; Skripconoka, V; Sanchez-Garavito, E; Xiao, H; Cabrera-Rivero, JL; Vargas-Vasquez, DE; Gao, M; Awad, M; Park, SK; Shim, TS; Suh, GY; Danilovits, M; Ogata, H; Kurve, A; Chang, J; Suzuki, K; Tupasi, T; Koh, WJ; Seaworth, B; Geiter, LJ; Wells, CD. Delamanid for multidrug-resistant pulmonary tuberculosis. *N Engl J Med* 2012, 366, 2151-2160.

[405] Skripconoka, V; Danilovits, M; Pehme, L; Tomson, T; Skenders, G; Kummik, T; Cirule, A; Leimane, V; Kurve, A; Levina, K; Geiter, LJ; Manissero, D; Wells, CD. Delamanid improves outcomes and reduces mortality for multidrug-resistant tuberculosis. *Eur Respir J* 2013, 41, 1393-1400.

[406] ClinicalTrials.gov. A phase 3, multicenter, randomized, double-blind, placebo-controlled parallel group trial to evaluate the safety and efficacy of delamanid administered orally as 200 mg total daily dose for six months in patients with pulmonary sputum culture-positive, multidrug-resistant tuberculosis. *Trial Identifier*: NCT01424670.

[407] Protopopova, M; Hanrahan, C; Nikonenko, B; Samala, R; Chen, P; Gearhart, J; Einck, L; Nacy, CA. Identification of a new antitubercular drug candidate, SQ109, from a combinatorial library of 1,2-ethylenediamines. *J Antimicrob Chemother* 2005, 56, 968-974.

[408] Nikonenko, BV; Protopopova, MN; Samala, R; Einck, L; Nacy, CA. Drug therapy of experimental TB: improved outcome by combining SQ109, a new diamine antibiotic with existing TB drugs. *Antimicrob Agents Chemother* 2007, 51, 1563-1565.

[409] Reddy, VM; Einck, L; Andries, K; Nacy, CA. In vitro interactions between new antitubercular drug candidates SQ109 and TMC 207. *Antimicrob Agents Chemother* 2010, 54, 2840-2846.

[410] Tahlan, K; Wilson, R; Kastrinsky, DB; Arora, K; Nair, V; Fischer, E; Barnes, SW; Walker, JR; Alland, D; Barry, CE 3rd; Boshoff, HI. SQ109 targets MmpL3, a membrane transporter of trehalose monomycolate

involved in mycolic acid donation to the cell wall core of *Mycobacterium tuberculosis*. *Antimicrob Agents Chemother* 2012, 56, 1797-1809.

[411] Wallis, RS; Jakubiec, W; Mitton-Fry, M; Ladutko, L; Campbell, S; Paige, D; Silvia, A; Miller, PF. Rapid ealuation in whole blood culture of regimens for XDR-TB containing PNU-100480 (Sutezolid), TMC207, PA-824, SQ109, and pyrazinamide. *PLoS One* 2012, 7, article no. e30479.

[412] Reddy, VM; Dubuisson, T; Einck, L; Wallis, RS; Jakubiec, W; Ladukto, L; Campbell, S; Nacy, CA. SQ109 and PNU-100480 interact to kill *Mycobacterium tuberculosis* in vitro. *J Antimicrob Chemother* 2012, 67, 1163-1166.

[413] ClinicalTrials.gov. A phase 2a trial to evaluate the extended early bactericidal activity, safety, tolerability, and pharmacokinetics of SQ109 in adult subjects with newly diagnosed, uncomplicated, smear-positive, pulmonary tuberculosis. *Trial Identifier*: NCT01218217

[414] Shaw, KJ; Barbachyn, MR. The oxazolidinones: past, present, and future. *Ann N Y Acad Sci* 2011, 1241, 48-70.

[415] Alffenaar, JW; vanAltena, R; Harmelink, IM; Filguera, P; Molenaar, E; Wessels, AM; van Soolingen, D; Kosterink, JG; Uges, DR; van der Werf, TS. Comparison of the pharmacokinetics of two dosage regimens of linezolid in multidrug-resistant and extensively drug-resistant tuberculosis patients. *Clin Pharmacokinet* 2010, 49, 559-565.

[416] Williams, KN; Stover, CK; Zhu, T; Tasneen, R; Tyagi, S; Grosset, JH; Nuermberger, E. Promising antituberculosis activity of the oxazolidinone PNU-100480 relative to that of linozolid in a murine model. *Antimicrob Agents Chemother* 2009, 53, 1314-1319.

[417] Williams, KN; Brickner, SJ; Stover, CK; Zhu, T; Ogden, A; Tasneen, R; Tyagi, S; Grosset, JH; Nuermberger, E. Addition of PNU-100480 to first-line drugs shortens the time needed to cure murine tuberculosis. *Am J Respir Crit Care Med* 2009, 180, 371-376.

[418] Wallis, RS; Jakubiec, W; Kumar, V; Bedarida, G; Silvia, A; Paige, D; Zhu, T; Mitton-Fry, M; Ladutko, L; Campbell, S; Miller, PF. Biomarker-assisted dose selection for safety and efficacy in early development of PNU-100480 for tuberculosis. *Antimicrob Agents Chemother* 2011, 55, 567-574.

[419] ClinicalTrials.gov. A phase-1, single center, double-blind, randomized, placebo-controlled, parallel-group study to assess the safety, tolerability and pharmacokinetics (including food effect) of ascending oral doses of

AZD5847 in healthy male subjects and female subjects of non-childbearing potential. *Trial Identifier*: NCT01037725.

[420] ClinicalTrials.gov. A phase-1, single center, double-blind, randomized, placebo-controlled, parallel-group, multiple ascending dose study to assess the safety, tolerability and pharmacokinetics of AZD5847 following oral administration to healthy male subjects and female subjects of non-childbearing potential. *Trial Identifier*: NCT01116258

[421] ClinicalTrials.gov. Randomized, open label, multiple dose phase 2a study of the early bactericidal activity of AZD5847 in adults with pulmonary tuberculosis. *Trial Identifier*: NCT01516203

[422] Makarov, V; Manina, G; Mikusova, K; Möllmann, U; Ryabova, O; Saint-Joanis, B; Dhar, N; Pasca, MR; Buroni, S; Lucarelli, AP; Milano, A; De Rossi, E; Belanova, M; Bobovska, A; Dianiskova, P; Kordulakova, J; Sala, C; Fullam, E; Schneider, P; McKinney, JD; Brodin, P; Christophe, T; Waddell, S; Butcher, P; Albrethsen, J; Rosenkrands, I; Brosch, R; Nandi, V; Bharath, S; Gaonkar, S; Shandil, RK; Balasubramanian, V; Balganesh, T; Tyagi, S; Grosset, J; Riccardi, G; Cole, ST. Benzothiazinones kill *Mycobacterium tuberculosis* by blocking arabinan synthesis. *Science* 2009, 324, 801-804.

[423] Pasca, MR; Degiacomi, G; Ribeiro, AL; Zara, F; De Mori, P; Heym, B; Mirrione, M; Brerra, R; Pagani, L; Pucillo, L; Troupioti, P; Makarov, V; Cole, ST; Riccardi, G. Clinical isolates of *Mycobacterium tuberculosis* in four European hospitals are uniformly susceptible to benzothiazinones. *Antimicrob Agents Chemother* 2010, 54, 1616-1618.

[424] Manina, G; Bellinzoni, M; Pasca, MR; Neres, J; Milano, A; Ribeiro, AL; Buroni, S; Skovierová, H; Dianišková, P; Mikušová, K; Marák, J; Makarov, V; Giganti, D; Haouz, A; Lucarelli, AP; Degiacomi, G; Piazza, A; Chiarelli, LR; De Rossi, E; Salina, E; Cole' ST; Alzari, PM; Riccardi, G. Biological and structural characterization of the *Mycobacterium smegmatis* nitroreductase NfnB, and its role in benzothiazinone resistance. *Mol Microbiol* 2010, 77, 1172-1185.

[425] Trefzer, C; Skovierová, H; Buroni, S; Bobovská, A; Nenci, S; Molteni, E; Pojer, F; Pasca, MR; Makarov, V; Cole, ST; Riccardi, G; Mikušová, K; Johnsson, K. Benzothiazinones are suicide inhibitors of mycobacterial decaprenylphosphoryl-β-d-ribofuranose 2'-oxidase DprE1. *J Am Chem Soc* 2012, 134, 912-915.

[426] Batt, SM; Jabeen, T; Bhowruth, V; Quill, L; Lund, PA; Eggeling, L; Alderwick, LJ; Fütterer, K; Besra, GS. Structural basis of inhibition of

Mycobacterium tuberculosis DprE1 by benzothiazinone inhibitors. *Proc Natl Acad Sci USA* 2012, 109, 11354-11359.

[427] Lechartier, B; Hartkoorn, RC; Cole, ST. In vitro combination studies of benzothiazinone lead compound BTZ043 against *Mycobacterium tuberculosis*. *Antimicrob Agents Chemother* 2012, 56, 5790-5793.

[428] Christophe, T; Christophe, T; Jackson, M; Jeon, HK; Fenistein, D; Contreras-Dominguez, M; Kim, J; Genovesio, A; Carralot, JP; Ewann, F; Kim, EH; Lee, SY; Kang, S; Seo, MJ; Park, EJ; Skovierová, H; Pham, H; Riccardi, G; Nam, JY; Marsollier, L; Kempf, M; Joly-Guillou, ML; Oh, T; Shin, WK; No, Z; Nehrbass, U; Brosch, R; Cole, ST; Brodin, P. High content screening identifies decaprenyl-phosphoribose 2' epimerase as a target for intracellular antimycobacterial inhibitors. *PLoS Pathog* 2009, 5, article no. e1000645.

[429] Ribeiro, AL; Degiacomi, G; Ewann, F; Buroni, S; Incandela, ML; Chiarelli, LR; Mori, G; Kim, J; Contreras-Dominguez, M; Park, YS; Han, SJ; Brodin, P; Valentini, G; Rizzi, M; Riccardi, G; Pasca, MR. Analogous mechanisms of resistance to benzothiazinones and dinitrobenzamides in *Mycobacterium smegmatis*. *PLoS One* 2011, 6, article no. e26675.

[430] Bogatcheva, E; Hanrahan, C; Chen, P; Gearhart, J; Sacksteder, K; Einck, L; Nacy, C; Protopopova, M. Discovery of dipiperidines as new antitubercular agents. *Bioorg Med Chem Lett* 2010, 20, 201-205.

[431] Bogatcheva, E; Hanrahan, C; Nikonenko, B; de los Santos, G; Reddy, V; Chen, P; Barbosa, F; Einck, L; Nacy, C; Protopopova, M. Identification of SQ609 as a lead compound from a library of dipiperidines. *Bioorg Med Chem Lett* 2011, 21, 5353-5357.

[432] Reddy, VM; Einck, L; Nacy, CA. In vitro antimycobacterial activities of capuramycin analogues. *Antimicrob Agents Chemother* 2008, 52, 719-721.

[433] Koga, T; Fukuoka, T; Doi, N; Harasaki, T; Inoue, H; Hotoda, H; Kakuta, M; Muramatsu, Y; Yamamura, N; Hoshi, M; Hirota, T. Activity of capuramycin analogues against *Mycobacterium tuberculosis*, *Mycobacterium avium* and *Mycobacterium intracellulare in vitro* and *in vivo*. *J Antimicrob Chemother* 2004, 54, 755-760

[434] Bogatcheva, E; Dubuisson, T; Protopopova, M; Einck, L; Nacy, CA; Reddy, VM. Chemical modification of capuramycins to enhance antibacterial activity. *J Antimicrob Chemother* 2011, 66, 578-587.

[435] Hirano, S; Ichikawa, S; Matsuda, A. Structure-activity relationship of truncated analogs of caprazamycins as potential anti-tuberculosis agents. *Bioorg Med Chem* 2008, 16, 5123-5133.

[436] http://www.tbdrugdiscovery.org/pdfs/TBDD, "2008 Update: The Lilly TB Drug Discovery Initiative begins work on new compounds to fill early-stage TB drug pipeline," 2008.

[437] Disratthakit, A; Doi, N. *In vitro* activities of DC-159a, a novel fluoroquinolone, against *Mycobacterium* species. *Antimicrob Agents Chemother* 2010, 54, 2684-2686.

[438] Sekiguchi, J; Disratthakit, A; Maeda, S; Doi, N. Characteristic resistance mechanism of *Mycobacterium tuberculosis* to DC-159a, a new respiratory quinolone. *Antimicrob Agents Chemother* 2011, 55, 3958-3960.

[439] Ahmad, Z; Minkowski, A; Peloquin, CA; Williams, KN; Mdluli, KE; Grosset, JH; Nuermberger, EL. Activity of the fluoroquinolone DC-159a in the initial and continuation phases of treatment of murine tuberculosis. *Antimicrob Agents Chemother* 2011, 55, 1781-1783.

[440] Deidda, D; Lampis, G; Fioravanti, R; Biava, M; Porretta, GC; Zanetti, S; Pompei, R. Bactericidal activities of the pyrrole derivative BM212 against multidrug-resistant and intramacrophagic *Mycobacterium tuberculosis* strains. *Antimicrob Agents Chemother* 1998, 42, 3035-3037.

[441] Biava, M; Porretta, GC; Poce, G; Supino, S; Deidda, D; Pompei, R; Molicotti, P; Manetti, F; Botta, M. Antimycobacterial agents. Novel diarylpyrrole derivatives of BM212 endowed with high activity toward *Mycobacterium tuberculosis* and low cytotoxicity. *J Med Chem* 2006, 49, 4946-4952.

[442] Biava, M; Porretta, GC; Poce, G; De Logu, A; Meleddu, R; De Rossi, E; Manetti, F; Botta, M. 1,5-Diaryl-2-ethyl pyrrole derivatives as antimycobacterial agents: design, synthesis, and microbiological evaluation. *Eur J Med Chem* 2009, 44, 4734-4738.

[443] Biava, M; Porretta, GC; Poce, G; Battilocchio, C; Alfonso, S; De Logu, A; Serra, N; Manetti, F; Botta, M. Identification of a novel pyrrole derivative endowed with antimycobacterial activity and protection index comparable to that of the current antitubercular drugs streptomycin and rifampin. *Bioorg Med Chem* 2010, 18, 8076-8084.

[444] La Rosa, V; Poce, G; Canseco, JO; Buroni, S; Pasca, MR; Biava, M; Raju, RM; Porretta, GC; Alfonso, S; Battilocchio, C; Javid, B; Sorrentino, F; Ioerger, TR; Sacchettini, JC; Manetti, F; Botta, M; De

Logu, A; Rubin, EJ; De Rossi, E. MmpL3 is the cellular target of the antitubercular pyrrole derivative BM212. *Antimicrob Agents Chemother* 2012, 56, 324-331.

[445] Grzegorzewicz, AE; Pham, H; Gundi, VA; Scherman, MS; North, EJ; Hess, T; Jones, V; Gruppo, V; Born, SE; Korduláková, J; Chavadi, SS; Morisseau, C; Lenaerts, AJ; Lee, RE; McNeil, MR; Jackson, M. Inhibition of mycolic acid transport across the *Mycobacterium tuberculosis* plasma membrane. *Nat Chem Biol* 2012, 8, 334-341.

[446] Maeda, K; Kosaka, H; Okami, Y; Umizawa, H. A new antibiotic, pyridomycin. *J Antibiot (Tokyo)* 1953, 6, 140.

[447] Shomura, T; Amano, S; Yoshida, J; Kojima, M. *Dactylosporangium fulvum* sp. nov. *Int J Syst Bacteriol* 1986, 36, 166-169.

[448] Hartkoorn, RC; Sala, C; Neres, J; Pojer, F; Magnet, S; Mukherjee, R; Uplekar, S; Boy-Röttger, S; Altmann, KH; Cole, ST. Towards a new tuberculosis drug: pyridomycin - nature's isoniazid. *EMBO Mol Med* 2012, 4, 1032-1042.

[449] Oliveira, JS; Pereira, JH; Canduri, F; Rodrigues, NC; de Souza, ON; de Azevedo, WF Jr; Basso, LA; Santos, DS. Crystallographic and pre-steady-state kinetics studies on binding of NADH to wild-type and isoniazid-resistant enoyl-ACP(CoA) reductase enzymes from *Mycobacterium tuberculosis*. *J Mol Biol* 2006, 359, 646-666.

[450] Villar, R; Vicente, E; Solano, B; Pérez-Silanes, S; Aldana, I; Maddry, JA; Lenaerts, AJ; Franzblau, SG; Cho, SH; Monge, A; Goldman, RC. *In vitro* and *in vivo* antimycobacterial acitivities of ketone and amide derivatives of quinoxaline 1,4-di-N-oxide. *J Antimicrob Chemother* 2008, 62, 547-554.

[451] Lilienkampf, A; Mao, J; Wan, B; Wang, Y; Franzblau, SG; Kozikowski, AP. Structure-activity relationships for a series of quinoline-based compounds against replicating and nonreplicating *Mycobacterium tuberculosis*. *J Med Chem* 2009, 52, 2109-2118.

[452] Huang, Q; Mao, J; Wan, B; Wang, Y; Brun, R; Franzblau, SG; Kozikowski, AP. Searching for new cures for tuberculosis: design, synthesis, and biological evaluation of 2-methylbenzothiazoles. *J Med Chem* 2009, 52, 6757-6767.

[453] Guo, S; Song, Y; Huang, Q; Yuan, H; Wan, B; Wang, Y; He, R; Beconi, MG; Franzblau, SG; Kozikowski, AP. Identification, synthesis, and pharmacological evaluation of tetrahydroindazole based ligands as novel antituberculosis agents. *J Med Chem* 2010, 53, 649-659.

[454] Saquib, M; Husain, I; Sharma, S; Yadav, G; Singh, VK; Sharma, SK; Shah, P; Siddiqi, MI; Kumar, B; Lal, J; Jain, GK; Srivastava, BS; Srivastava, R; Shaw, AK. 2,3-dideoxy hex-2-enopyranosid-4-uloses as promising new anti-tubercular agents: design, synthesis, biological evaluation and SAR studies. *Eur J Med Chem* 2011, 46, 2217-2223.

[455] Upadhayaya, RS; Shinde, PD; Kadam, SA; Bawane, AN; Sayyed, AY; Kardile, RA; Gitay, PN; Lahore, SV; Dixit, SS; Földesi, A; Chattopadhyaya, J. Synthesis and antimycobacterial activity of prodrugs of indeno[2,1-c]quinoline derivatives. *Eur J Med Chem* 2011, 46, 1306-1324.

[456] Forge, D; Cappoen, D; Laurent, J; Stanicki, D; Mayence, A; Huang, TL; Verschaeve, L; Huygen, K; Vanden Eynde, JJ. 1,4-diarylpiperazines and analogs as anti-tubercular agents: synthesis and biological evaluation. *Eur J Med Chem* 2012, 49, 95-101.

[457] Cappoen, D; Jacobs, J; Nguyen Van, T; Claessens, S; Diels, G; Anthonissen, R; Einarsdottir, T; Fauville, M; Verschaeve, L; Huygen, K; De Kimpe, N. Straightforward palladium-mediated synthesis and biological evaluation of benzo[j]phenanthridine-7,12-diones as anti-tuberculosis agents. *Eur J Med Chem* 2012, 48, 57-68.

[458] Almansour, AI; Suresh Kumar, R; Arumugam, N; Sriram, D. A solvent free, four-component synthesis and 1,3-dipolar cycloaddition of 4(H)-pyrans with nitrile oxides: synthesis and discovery of antimycobacterial activity of enantiomerically pure 1,2,4-oxadiazoles. *Eur J Med Chem* 2012, 53, 416-423.

[459] Rudra, S; Yadav, A; Raja Rao, AV; Srinivas, AS; Pandya, M; Bhateja, P; Mathur, T; Malhotra, S; Rattan, A; Salman, M; Mehta, A; Cliffe, IA; Das, B. Synthesis and antibacterial activity of potent heterocyclic oxazolidinones and the identification of RBx 8700. *Bioorg Med Chem Lett* 2007, 17, 6714-6719.

[460] Gonçalves, RS; Kaiser, CR; Lourenço, MC; Bezerra, FA; de Souza, MV; Wardell, JL; Wardell, SM; Henriques, Md; Costa, T. Mefloquine-oxazolidine derivatives, derived from mefloquine and arenecarbaldehydes: *in vitro* activity including against the multidrug-resistant tuberculosis strain T113. *Bioorg Med Chem* 2012, 20, 243-248.

Index

D

E

F

G

H

I

J

T

U

V

W

Y